LEUCOCYTE DEPLETION OF BLOOD COMPONENTS

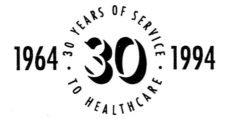

Presented with the compliments
of

KIMAL

Scientific Products Ltd.

in
Commemoration of the
30th Anniversary.

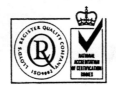

Leucocyte Depletion of Blood Components

CLAES F. HÖGMAN
editor

VU University Press
Amsterdam 1994

VU University Press is an imprint of:
VU Boekhandel/Uitgeverij bv
De Boelelaan 1105
1081 HV Amsterdam
The Netherlands

tel.   +31(0)20 6444355
fax   +31(0)20 6462719

isbn   90-5383-275-0
nugi   743

Layout: Sjoukje Rienks, Amsterdam
Cover design: Neroc Special Services, Amsterdam
Printed by: Wilco, Amersfoort

Preface

On 9th July 1988, in London before the XXth Congress of the International Society of Blood Transfusion, the first International Workshop on the Role of Leucocyte Depletion in Blood Transfusion Practice was organized. The Conference was held under the chairmanship of Dr. B. Brozovic and sponsored by Asahi Medical Co. Ltd, Tokyo, Japan. The Proceedings were published by Blackwell Scientific Publications in 1989 with Dr. Brozovic as editor.

The role of leucocytes in transfusion medicine has continued to stay in focus of interest during the six years that have passed since the time of the workshop. Much progress has been made and it was felt that a second workshop would be well motivated to summarize the present status of the item. Like the previous time a Workshop arranged for interested scientists in Transfusion Medicine is being arranged on the eve of the Congress of the International Society of Blood Transfusion, this time on 1st July 1994 in Amsterdam. Instead of proceedings published after the conference it has been decided to summarize the data in a book printed closely before the workshop to be distributed to the participants and, after the conference, to others interested. Contributions from invited speakers as well as poster presenters have been included in the publication.

I wish to express my warm thanks to Mr. N. Saijo and his colleagues of Asahi Medical GmbH, Frankfurt, Germany, Mr. John deMullet of JR International Consultancy, Bolton, England, and the staff of VU University Press, Amsterdam for taking care of all practical aspects of this workshop and publication, as well as to all speakers for excellent collaboration.

Uppsala 31st March, 1994
CLAES F. HÖGMAN

Contents

Leucocyte Depletion of Blood Components – Present Trends and the Future. An Introduction

1 | C.F. Högman

In the 1970s leucocytes gained increased interest in blood component therapy. It was known that they could immunize a transfusion recipient, but it came as a surprise that they could also improve graft survival in kidney transplantation. Programmes for systematic pretransplant transfusions were developed. Later more effective pharmaceutical immunosuppression made it less common to use blood transfusion for improvement of kidney graft survival, although recent studies have clearly demonstrated the beneficial role of blood transfusion when the donor and recipient share at least one HLA-DR antigen (Lagaaij et al. 1989). A potentially negative effect of this immunomodulatory capacity of blood transfusion may be the cause of an increased incidence of bacterial, postoperative complications (Jensen et al. 1992) and cancer recurrence, probably mainly related to factors in donor leucocytes.

Transfusion-associated graft-versus-host disease (TA-GVHD) in immunocompetent persons is a rare but dreaded complication with high mortality. The major reason is believed to be that the recipient does not reject transfused, viable leucocytes, when the donor is homozygous for one of the recipient's haplotypes, causing a graft which combats the host. However, this combination of donor-recipient HLA-DR haplotypes – in a US population 1 in 7174 for unrelated donors and 1 in 475 for first-degree relatives – has been estimated to occur much more frequently than the actual observation of TA-GVHD. Recent data indicate that an active mechanism exists in immunocompetent individuals which inhibits the graft versus host reaction (Van der Mast et al. 1994).

The development of improved apheresis techniques in the 1970s made it possible to prepare granulocyte concentrates which were used to combat bacterial septicaemia in severely neutropenic patients. But effective antibiotics and the great efforts needed to obtain sufficiently large doses of granulocytes brought leucocyte transfusion more or less out of fashion in adult patients in the 80s. Recently, the use of growth factors submitted to the donor makes it possible to increase the therapeutical efficacy which may give this way of treatment a come-back.

Another matter for much discussion in the 1970s was the participation of leucocytes in microaggregates which, after massive transfusions, were considered to impair pulmonary oxygenation by blocking of lung capillaries. As a consequence removal of buffy coat, mainly as a measure to decrease the contents of microaggregates, was introduced as a routine procedure in some countries (Prins et al. 1980). Microaggregate filters were used for the same purpose at large scale in others; they were later found useful in the reduction of the leucocyte contents in red cell concentrates (Wenz 1983).

At the time of the First International Workshop on the Role of Leucocyte Depletion in Blood Transfusion Practice (Brozovic 1989) the role of posttransfusion HLA immunization in the recipient causing refractoriness to platelet transfusion had been identified as an important medical hazard. Several procedures were developed for leucocyte depletion of red cell and platelet concentrates. Two principles for leucocyte removal dominated, either each alone or both in combination: centrifugation and removal of the buffy coat, or passing the blood through special leucocyte removing filters. Both methods have been further developed and improved. Removal of buffy coat has the advantage that it can be easily incorporated in an automated blood component routine process at limited expense in materials and labour. The least dense white cells, i.e. lymphocytes and monocytes, are removed more effectively than the more dense granulocytes (Nakajo et al. 1993). Storage in the cold improves removal, resulting in a mean leucocyte content of about 0.1-0.5×10^9 leucocytes per unit of red cells with the best procedures (Kretschmer et al. 1988). This reduces the incidence of febrile transfusion reactions and seems to reduce but not eliminate HLA immunization (Leikola and Myllylä 1990). Preparation of platelets from buffy coat instead of from platelet rich plasma fits in logistically extremely well with the removal of buffy coat from red cells. But what is its actual benefit in today's medicine? Preparation of platelet concentrates from buffy coats frequently results in smaller leucocyte contamination. Lower platelet yields have been observed in some investigations, satisfactory ones in others. Apheresis techniques for the preparation of platelet concentrates have also been much improved with respect to low contents of leucocytes.

When shall the leucocytes be removed – in direct conjunction with blood donation, at blood component preparation after some hours holding at room temperature, or bedside at transfusion? A beneficial effect of leucocytes in the freshly collected blood has been demonstrated under experimental conditions, reducing, by phagocytosis, the contents of contaminating bacteria (Högman et al. 1991), although their role as 'safety factors' in the production of blood components is still unknown. Leucocytes may host viable viruses, CMV in particular (Gilbert et al. 1989), and bacteria (Högman et al. 1992). Thus, leucocyte removal seems to be a way of making blood components safer with respect to the transfer of infectious agents, but an optimal procedure may need some hours of holding at 22°C.

Leucocyte removing filters have gradually been improved with respect to their capacity to achieve leucocyte depletion. It is possible to obtain 3-4 log reduction of the initial leucocyte content, thus resulting in a leucocyte dose well below 5-10×10^6 white cells per transfusion of red cells or platelets, suggested as the borderline below which HLA immunization is very unlikely (Leikola and Myllylä 1990). Bedside leucofiltration in connection with transfusion of red cells has become a standard procedure, when it is highly desirable to avoid HLA immunization (Vakkila and Myllylä 1987), and has been reported to give reaction free transfusions in multiply transfused patients (Sirchia et al. 1990). However, filters differ with respect to their capacity to remove leucocytes (Pietersz et al. 1993) and failures may occur depending on the nature of the filter and the technique of filtration. An important problem is the reliability of the leucodepletion procedure; one failure may be enough to initiate primary immunization in a non-transfused patient.

The methods to detect small numbers of white cells have been gradually improved and recommendations concerning useful techniques have been given by an international group of experts (Rebulla and Dzik 1994). Commonly, the quality of red cell or platelet concentrates with respect to their contents of leucocytes is presented as total number of remaining leucocytes without taking notice of what types of leucocytes they are. For primary immunization the presence of antigen presenting cells, carrying HLA class II antigens, is important, whereas for boosting an already existing immunization, cells such as granulocytes and platelets, carrying class I antigens, may be equally active.

Irradiation of mononuclear cells with ultraviolet light is a possibility to abolish the capacity of lymphocytes to stimulate to DNA synthesis in a mixed lymphocyte culture (Lindahl-Kiessling and Säfwenberg 1971). Methods have been developed to use this principle for reducing the immunogenicity of blood components (Kahn et al. 1985, Pamphilon et al. 1989). What is the role of UV irradiation in blood transfusion practice today?

Experimental studies have shown that for the occurrence of HLA immunization there is a need of an accessory signal from the antigen presenting cell (Meryman, review, 1989). However, the capacity to produce this signal is lost within 14 days when the blood is stored at refrigerator temperature (Mincheff et al. 1993). If thus the presence of viable, HLA class II antigen carrying donor leucocytes is necessary for obtaining HLA immunization, is primary immunization then avoided when such cells are strongly reduced or have lost viability, even in the presence of class I carrying cells? Should we put moderately leucocyte-reduced red cell units in quarantine for some weeks before using them, in order to further decrease their immunogenicity? What quality is required in previously non-transfused infants to avoid immunization? The degree of freedom from lymphocytes, monocytes, dendritic cells and granulocytes that is needed in blood components in order to avoid immunomodulatory effects in the recipients, seems to be a matter for further elucidation.

In conclusion, the positive and negative roles of allogeneic leucocytes, particularly as contaminating living and normally functioning cells, but maybe also as cell fragments or soluble membrane substances, present in red cell and platelet concentrates, and the importance and possibilities to remove them, are still matters of great interest. To what extent do we need to deplete our blood components from leucocytes? Are our present methods for preparation of blood components optimal with regard to cost-effectiveness? If not, what shall we do to improve them? What is the theoretical evidence and the clinical experience?

It is my hope that this workshop will summarize current knowledge on leucocyte depletion of blood components in an interesting and profitable way and guide us toward further improvements in the future.

References

Brozovic B. (ed.) (1989) *The role of leucocyte depletion in blood transfusion practice,* Blackwell Scientific Publications, Oxford.

Gilbert G.L., Hayes K., Hudson I.L., James J. (1989) Prevention of transfusion-acquired cytomegalovirus infection in infants by blood filtration to remove leukocytes, *Lancet* i: 1228-1231.

Högman C.F., Gong J., Eriksson L., Hambraeus A., Johansson C.S. (1991) White cells protect donor blood against bacterial contamination, *Transfusion* 31: 620-626.

Högman C.F., Gong J., Hambraeus A., Johansson C.S., Eriksson L. (1992) The role of white cells in the transmission of Yersinia enterocolitica in blood components, *Transfusion* 32: 654-657.

Jensen L.S., Andersen A.J., Christiansen P.M., Hokland P., Juhl C.O., Madsen G., Mortensen J., Møller-Nielsen C., Hanberg-Sørensen F., Hokland M. (1992) Postoperative infection and natural killer cell function following blood transfusion in patients undergoing colorectal surgery, *Br. J. Surg.* 79: 513-516.

Kretschmer V., Kahn-Blouki K., Biermann E., Söhngen D., Eckle R. (1988) Improvement of blood component quality – automatic separation of blood components in a new bag system, *Infusionstherapie* 15: 232-239.

Lagaaij E.L., Henneman I.P.H., Ruigrok M., De Haan M.W., Persijn G.G., Termijtelen A., Hendriks G.F.J., Weimar W., Claas F.H.J., Van Rood J.J. (1989) Effect of one-HLA-DR-Antigen-matched and completely HLA-DR-mismatched blood transfusions on survival of heart and kidney allografts, *N. Engl. J. Med.* 321: 701-705.

Leikola J., Myllylä G. (1990) The clinical use of red blood cell components, in: Summers S.H., Smith D.M., Agranenko V.A. (eds.) *Transfusion Therapy,* American Association of Blood Banks, Arlington, VA, pp. 1-25.

Lindahl-Kiessling K., Säfwenberg J. (1971) Inability of UV-irradiated lymphocytes to stimulate allogeneic cells in mixed lymphocyte culture, *Int. Arch. Allergy* 41: 670-678.

Meryman H.T. (1989) Transfusion-induced alloimmunization and immuno-suppression and the effects of leukocyte depletion, *Trans. Med. Rev.* 3: 180-193.

Mincheff M.S., Meryman H.T., Kapoor V., Alsop P. Wötzel M. (1993) Blood transfusion and immunomodulation: a possible mechanism, *Vox Sang.* 65: 18-24.

Nakajo S., Chiba S., Takahashi T.A., Sekiguchi S. (1993) Comparison of a 'top and bottom' system with a conventional quadruple-bag system for blood-component preparation and storage, in: Sekighuchi S. (ed.) *Clinical Application of Leukocyte Depletion,* Blackwell Scientific Publications, Oxford, pp. 18-30.

Pamphilon D.H., Corbin S. Saunders J., Tandy N. (1989) Application of ultraviolet light in the preparation of platelet concentrates, *Transfusion* 29: 378-383.

Pietersz R.N.I, Steneker I., Reesink H.W. (1993) Prestorage leukocyte depletion of blood products in a closed system, *Trans. Med. Rev.* 7: 17-24.

Prins H.K., De Bruijn J.C.G.H., Henrichs H.P.J., Loos J.A. (1980) Prevention of microaggregate formation by removal of 'buffy coats', *Vox Sang.* 39: 48-51.

Rebulla P., Dzik W.H. (1994) Multicenter evaluation of methods for counting residual white cells in leukocyte-depleted red blood cells, *Vox Sang.* 66: 25-32.

Sirchia G., Wenz B., Rebulla P., Parravicini A., Carnelli V., Bertolini F. (1990) Removal of white cells from red cells by transfusion through a new filter, *Transfusion* 30: 30-33.

Vakkila J., Myllylä G. (1987) Amount and type of leukocytes in 'leukocyte-free' red cell and platelet concentrates, *Vox Sang.* 53: 76-82.

Van der Mast B.J., Hornstra N., Ruigrok M.B., Claas F.H.J, Van Rood J.J., Lagaaij E.L. (1994) Transfusion-associated graft-versus-host disease in immunocompetent patients: a self-protective mechanism, *Lancet* 343: 753-757.

Wenz B. (1983) Microaggregate blood filtration and the febrile transfusion reaction, *Transfusion* 23: 95-98.

Mechanism of Alloimmunization to HLA Antigen

2 | H.T. Meryman and M.S. Mincheff

Alloimmunization against HLA antigens is a common occurrence in transfused patients. We have previously reviewed data from 7 clinical studies in which 79 of 161 (50%) of patients receiving unfiltered red cells or platelets became alloimmunized (Meryman 1989). The rate in individual studies varied from 6% to 93%, implying that transfusion-induced alloimmunization can be readily influenced by other factors, among which are probably extent of leucocyte contamination, age of the blood products, extent of HLA antigen disparity and the immune status of the recipient. The development of alloimmunization appears to be independent of the number of transfusions administered and the patients tend to become immunized early in the treatment course (Bonacossa 1990). If alloimmunization does not develop within the first few weeks of transfusions, it rarely develops later despite repeated transfusions (Bonacossa 1990).

Evidence has accumulated that the presence of leucocytes in the donor blood contributes to the likelihood of alloimmunization since reducing the numbers of transfused leucocytes results in a reduced frequency of sero-conversion (Meryman 1989, Claas et al. 1981).

Two types of major histocompatibility complex (MHC) molecules have been described: Class I is present on most cells of the body, although expression varies widely and is typically highest on hemopoietic elements. The Class I MHC is recognized by the CD8 (cytotoxic) T cell. Class II is expressed primarily by 'professional' antigen-presenting cells (APCs) which include dendritic cells, B cells, macrophages, and monocytes. The Class II MHC is recognized by the CD4 (helper) T Cell, a primary function of which is the secretion of interleukin 2 (IL-2) which is required for the proliferation of CD8 cells, B cells and the CD4 cells themselves.

Experimental evidence indicates that the antigen-presenting cells in the transfused blood must be intact and viable in order to initiate alloimmunization (Deeg 1989, Andreu et al. 1990, Mincheff et al. 1993). The ability to induce an immune response in vitro can be decreased or eliminated by ultraviolet-B (UV-B) (Schlichter et al. 1987) or gamma irradiation (Mincheff et al. 1989), unprotected freezing (Anonymous 1989), pressurization (Meryman H.T., Mincheff M., unpublished) or 4°C storage (Mincheff et al. 1993). The critical role of the Class II-bearing APC is further supported by the observation that HLA DR-identical transfusions do not alloimmunize (Meryman 1989) and the incidence of immunization is substantially reduced when DR-haplotype-identical transfusions are administered, regardless of mismatch of the Class I phenotype (Anonymous 1989). It also appears that presentation of Class I MHC antigens in the absence of Class II does not lead to alloimmunization, perhaps because of the absence of the IL-2 secretion by activated CD4 cells, and that Class II-bearing cells are the probable source of transfusion-induced alloimmunization.

On the other hand, an accumulation of clinical data from patients receiving leucocyte-depleted red cells and platelets continues to reveal a significant incidence of alloimmunization despite depletion of leucocytes (Sniecinski et al. 1988). It is not known whether this means that even leucocyte contamination of the order of 10^4 cells is still sufficient to immunize, whether the large quantity of Class I antigen contributed by platelets may be a factor or whether there are other sources of immunization.

Virtually all adaptive immune responses involve clonal expansion of naive CD4+ T cells. The ability to drive this process is the defining characteristic of a competent APC. It is now generally agreed that Class II-bearing APCs internalize protein antigens from their environment and degrade them in intracellular acid compartments (Unanue and Allen 1987). The resulting peptides are expressed at the cell surfaces in conjunction with the Class II MHC which is synthesized within these cells.

More than 20 years ago Bretscher and Cohn proposed the 'two signal hypothesis' for lymphocyte activation, which dealt with the ongoing need to maintain self tolerance in the case of B-cell hypermutation (Bretscher and Cohn 1970). They suggested that a B cell must receive two consecutive signals in order to be activated: Signal 1 from the antigen and Signal 2 from a second cell specific for the same antigen, e.g. a T helper cell (Unanue and Allen 1987). Although this model was originally proposed to explain activation of B cells, its principles are also valid for T cells (Cohn 1989).

The Class II MHC-peptide complex is recognized by a receptor molecule on the CD4 (helper) T-cell (TCR) (Brown et al. 1988). This interaction results in intracellular events within the CD4 cell such as mobilization of calcium and phosphorus, generation of diacyl glycerol, stimulation of protein kinase C and expression on the cell surface of the interleukin-2 (IL-2) receptor (Mueller et al. 1989). However, IL-2, which CD4 cells require to proliferate, is not secreted at this stage (Mueller et al. 1989). Secretion of IL-2 requires an additional accessory signal which appear to include surface molecules on the APCs and their respective ligands on the CD4 cells (Mincheff and Meryman 1989). To initiate an immunogenic response, therefore, both the MHC-peptide signal and the accessory signal must be expressed by the APC and recognized by CD4 T cells (Schlichter et al. 1987, Mincheff and Meryman 1989, Mincheff et al. 1993).

The provision of the accessory signal is essential for the secretion of IL-2 by CD4 cells and for the subsequent proliferation of activated T and B-cells. Despite presentation of MHC-peptide and its recognition by the CD4 T-cell receptor (TCR), no further immunogenic response will be seen in the absence of this additional signal. On the other hand T-cells that recognize the MHC-peptide signal but do not receive the accessory signal become unresponsive (anergic) to the specific MHC-peptide complex presented, even though subsequent encounters might involve a complete signal including both MHC-peptide and the accessory signal (Jenkins and Schwartz 1987, Jenkins et al. 1988, Schwartz 1989, Nossal 1989). We have proposed (Mincheff et al. 1993) that T cell anergy may be responsible for the immunosuppression induced by transfusions.

Crystallographic evidence (Bjorkman et al. 1987a, Bjorkman et al. 1987b) reveals that the MHC molecules contain two immunoglobulin-like domains proximal to the membrane. Distal to the membrane are eight beta-strands and two long alpha helices that form the bottom and the sides of the peptide-binding groove. Most allele-specific residues lie on, or between these helices and potentially affect the shape of the binding site. Peptides bind to the groove by conserved pockets at its ends while the middle of the peptide is less constrained by MHC and more exposed for direct interaction with the T cell receptor. Differences in length and aminoacid sequence of the peptides are accommodated by 'bulging' away from the groove (Guo et al. 1992). Different peptides may bind to one and the same MHC molecule thus creating different antigenic specificities. An alloantigen, consequently, is a binary complex of an MHC molecule and numerous antigen-derived (Class II) or endogenous (Class I) peptides and the high frequency of alloreactive T cells in vitro comes from the fact that the alloresponse is in fact always polyclonal.

Since T cells recognize various binary complexes of 'alloMHC + X^1, X^2, ..., X^N, where Xs are different donor- or recipient-derived peptides, both alloimmunization and immunosuppression are polyclonal. On the other hand similarity between an $MHC^A + X^1$ and an $MHC^B + X^2$ binary complex is possible. This implies that alloimmunization/immunosuppression achieved by a single blood transfusion may cover multiple specificities.

We have also shown that, during storage, lymphomononuclear cells progressively lose their ability to costimulate, and cells isolated from blood stored for 14 or more days are no longer immunogenic in vitro despite the continued presence of surface MHC (Mincheff et al. 1993). This leads us to predict not only that stored blood would not alloimmunize but that it would immunosuppress.

Incompetent APCs presenting only the MHC-peptide signal are not the only potential agents for the induction of T cell anergy. B cells also function as antigen-presenting cells, expressing both Class I and Class II MHC. However, B cells are constitutively incapable of expressing the accessory signal and are therefore potential initiators of T cell anergy in the absence of alloimmunization. This is consistent with the general impression that transfusions either alloimmunize or immunosuppress.

On the basis of these observations, we have initiated a clinical study to determine whether patients with negative HLA antibody screens receiving only aged, unfiltered red cells will alloimmunize. The study will also investigate whether patients initially receiving only stored cells will have been sufficiently immunosuppressed to prevent alloimmunization by subsequent fresh, unfiltered transfusions.

One exception to the general rule that the presence of viable leucocytes in a transfusion can induce alloimmunization while their removal will prevent it appears to be transfusions to bone marrow transplant recipients. We (Braine et al., in preparation) have recently completed a study which was designed to determine whether the few immunizations still seen following filtration of platelets could be prevented by more aggressive leucodepletion using elutriation. Surprisingly, a high incidence of alloimmunization was found in both the filtration (29%) and the elutriation (21%) arms of the study. Further analysis of the data revealed that all of the alloimmunizations occurred in patients receiving marrow allografts while no immunizations occurred in autograft recipients, even in the control group. Marrow transplants, therefore, represent a special case in which the marrow ablation inhibits an immune response to transfusions. In allografted patients, the immunization is apparently induced by the donor marrow. The mechanism for this may be that described above wherein APCs in the donor marrow activate recipient T and B cells which have survived the marrow ablation and continue to function until hematopoietic reconstitution with donor cells takes place. This speculation is supported by the fact that, in our study, the presence of antibody in immunized allograft recipients was always transitory, persisting for only a few weeks in all cases, unlike the usual experience wherein antibodies resulting from transfusion-induced immunization can often persist for more than a year. Alternatively, alloimmunity may be transferred via B cells from the marrow of donors who have been previously transfused although, in our study, there were patients who received bone marrow from donors who had not been previously transfused or exposed to foreign HLA through pregnancy.

In summary, transfusion induced alloimmunization appears to result from the recognition by recipient T cells of foreign MHC-peptide on viable donor antigen presenting cells. The depletion of contaminating leucocytes by filtration of red cells or platelets would therefore clearly be expected to reduce the incidence of alloimmunization.

Immunogenesis requires that CD4 cells receive both an initial MHC-peptide signal and a second, accessory signal. Inhibition of the accessory signal by UVB, by blood storage or by other modalities can block alloimmunization and perhaps lead to immunosuppression through T cell anergy induced either by such 'compromised' APCs or by B cells.

Bone marrow transplant recipients are an exception. Autograft recipients are not immunized by unfiltered transfusions, allograft recipients will immunize despite filtration.

From the practical standpoint, for patients in whom alloimmunization is clinically undesirable, leucocyte-depletion should be mandatory. However, transfusing only red cells that are two or more weeks old may replace filtration. Leucodepletion of any blood products may be unnecessary for marrow autograft recipients and ineffective for marrow allograft recipients.

References

Andreu G., Boccaccio C., Lecrubier C., Fretault J., Coursaget J., LeGuen J.P., Oleggini M., Fournell J.J., Samama M. (1990) Ultraviolet irradiation of platelet concentrates: Feasibility in transfusion practice, *Transfusion* 30: 401.

Anonymous (1989) Effect of one-HLA-DR-antigen-matched and completely HLA-DR-mismatched blood transfusions on survival of heart and kidney allografts, *New Engl. J. Med.* 321: 701.

Bjorkman P.J., Saper M.A., Samraoui B., Bennett W.S., Strominger J.L., Wiley D.C. (1987a) Structure of the human class I histocompatibility antigen, HLA-2, *Nature* 329: 506.

Bjorkman P.J., Saper M.A., Samraoui B., Bennett W.S., Strominger J.L., Wiley D.C. (1987b) The foreign antigen binding site and the T cell recognition regions of class I histocompatibility antigens, *Nature* 329: 512.

Bonacossa I.A. (1990) Alloimmunization as a problem for platelet transfusion, *Transf. Med. Reviews* 4: 144.

Braine H.G., Meryman H.T. et al. (in preparation) Transfusion-induced alloimmunization in bone-marrow transplant recipients.

Bretscher P., Cohn M. (1970) A theory of self-nonself discrimination, *Science* 169: 1042.

Brown J., Jardetzky T., Saper M.A., Samraoui B., Bjorkman P.J., Wiley D.C. (1988) A hypothetical model of the foreign antigen binding site of class II histocompatibility molecules, *Nature* 332: 845.

Claas F.H.J., Smeenk R.T.J., Schmidt R., Van Steenbrugge G.J., Eernisse J.G. (1981) Alloimmunization against the MHC antigens after platelet transfusions is due to contaminating leucocytes in the platelets, *Exp. Hematol.* 9: 84.

Cohn M. (1989) The apriori principles which govern immune responsiveness, in: 'Cellular Basis of Immune Modulation', AR Liss, New York, p. 11

Deeg H.J. (1989) Transfusion with a tan - Prevention of alloimmunization by ultraviolet irradiation, *Transfusion* 29: 450.

Guo H.C., Jardetzky T.S., Garrett T.P.J., Lane S.L., Strominger J.L., Wiley D.C. (1992) Different length peptides bind to HLA-Aw68 similarly at their ends but bulge out in the middle, *Nature* 360: 364.

Jenkins M.K., Ashwell J.D., Schwartz R.H. (1988) Allogeneic non-T spleen cells restore the responsiveness of normal T cell clones stimulated with antigen and chemically modified antigen presenting cells, *J. Immunol.* 140: 3324.

Jenkins M.K., Schwartz R.H. (1987) Antigen presentation by chemically modified splenocytes induces antigen-specific T cell unresponsiveness in vitro and in vivo, *J. Exp. Med.* 165: 302.

Meryman H.T. (1989) Transfusion-induced alloimmunization and immunosuppression and the effects of leucocyte depletion, *Transf. Med. Rev.* 3: 180.

Mincheff M.S., Meryman H.T. (1989) Induction of primary mixed leucocyte reactions with ultraviolet B or chemically modified stimulator cells, *Transplantation* 48: 1052.

Mincheff M.S., Meryman H.T., Kapoor V., Alsop P., Wotzel M. (1993) Blood transfusion and immunomodulation: a possible mechanism, *Vox Sang.* 65: 18.

Mueller D.L., Jenkins M.K., Schwartz R.H. (1989) An accessory cell-derived costimulatory signal acts independently of protein kinase C activation to allow T cell proliferation and prevent the induction of unresponsiveness, *J. Immunol.* 142: 2617.

Nossal G.J.V. (1989) Immunologic tolerance: collaboration between antigen and lymphokines, *Science* 245: 147.

Schlichter S.J., Deeg H.J., Kennedy M.S. (1987) Prevention of platelet alloimmunization in dogs with systemic cyclosporine and by UV-B irradiation or cyclosporine-loading of donor platelets, *Blood* 62: 815.

Schwartz, R.H. (1989) Acquisition of immunologic self-tolerance, *Cell* 57: 1073.

Sniecinski I., O'Donnell M.R., Nowicki B., Hill L.R. (1988) Prevention of refractoriness and HLA-alloimmunization using filtered blood products, *Blood* 71: 1402.

Unanue E., Allen P.M. (1987) The basis for the immunoregulatory role of macrophages and other accessory cells, *Science* 236: 551.

Positive and Negative Effects of Transfused Leucocytes

3 | A. Brand

Negative effects of leucocyte-depletion

Leucocyte-depletion of red cell and platelet transfusions emerged in the seventies to reduce the formation of HLA-antibodies. In the past decade efforts were made to extend the application for leucocyte-depleted blood products. The question whether leucocyte-depletion also could have negative effects on transfusion therapy - except increasing the costs - was hardly addressed. It is, due to lacking data, difficult to give the possible negative aspects of leucocyte-depletion a serious consideration.

Transplantation tolerance
Opelz and others observed an increased incidence of rejection of cadaver kidney grafts when patients had not received pre-transplantation blood transfusions (Opelz et al. 1973). The mechanism how pretransplantation blood transfusions protect against the allograft rejection is still not completely understood. The following characteristics were identified: one to three transfusates (whole blood, buffy-coats, red cell concentrates or platelets) containing approximately 0.5-1.5×10^9 leucocytes induced this immunosuppressive effect. Filtered red cell transfusions and leucocyte depleted platelet transfusions had no beneficial effect on graft survival (Persijn et al. 1979). Clinical studies with in-vitro follow up evaluation showed a dualistic effect on the immune response depending on the degree of MHC sharing between donor and recipient. Haplotype or at least HLA-DR-shared transfusions decreased the cytotoxic precursor cells against the transfusion donor in contrast to DR-mismatched transfusions (Van Twuijer et al. 1992).

DR-matched pretransplantation blood transfusions were in contrast to DR-mismatched transfusions associated with a reduced number of rejection episodes after subsequent kidney or heart transplantation (Lagaay et al. 1989).

Crohn's disease
The above mentioned immunosuppressive effects of blood transfusions on allograft rejection might be beneficial in auto-immune diseases as well. Patients suffering from immune-mediated diseases do not receive blood transfusions on a regular basis.

An exception are patients with Crohn's disease not responding to immunosuppressive treatment. Five retrospective studies compared transfused and non-transfused patients. Williams et al. (1991) studied 60 patients and found a significant reduction at five years in the transfused (19% recurrence) versus the non-transfused (59%) group. The localization of disease in the two groups was however different. Non-transfused patients had more often terminal ileal disease and transfused patients more small bowel diseases. Peters et al. (1989) compared multiple transfused with limited transfused patients with significant less recurrence in multi transfused patients. Scott et al. (1991) found in a large study that there was only a delay in recurrence in transfused patients. At 8 years post-surgery, there was no difference anymore. The largest retrospective study in 261 patients found no difference between the transfused and non-transfused patients (Post et al. 1992). The last study (Silvis et al. 1993) conducted in 148 patients found no difference in relapse incidence in the overall group of 62 males and 86 females. In this study parous women had the worst prognosis compared to non-parous females and males.

After perioperative transfusions parous females had a similar prognosis as non-parous females and males. In fact from none of the studies conclusions can be drawn as blood transfusions were significantly associated with all parameters for more severe disease such as duration and type of surgery, length of specimen removed, preoperative haemoglobin and perioperative blood loss. More relapses would be expected in this group. Even the observation that there is no difference in recurrence may be a reason to investigate the role of transfusions in patients with Crohn's disease.

As leucocytes are the major candidate to mediate a possible immune suppressive effect, leucocyte-depletion might be deleterious in case of perioperative transfusions for patients with Crohn's disease.

Graft Versus Leukaemia (GVL)
It was observed that transplanted leukaemia patients showed an improved disease free survival (DFS) after allogeneic marrow compared to syngeneic or autologous marrow transplantation. GVL is in some studies associated with graft versus host disease and is presumably mediated by immune competent allogeneic T cells directed against leukaemia associated antigens.

In 1989 Tucker retrospectively analysed two groups of patients with acute myeloid leukaemia (AML) transfused with standard (STD, N=19) or leucocyte-depleted (LP, N=17) red cells and platelet transfusions. Receivers of STD transfusions had a better DFS (50% at 3 years) compared to a low DFS in LP transfused patients (9% at 3 years). Standard platelet transfusions contained a huge amount of white cells ($5x10^9$) whereas LP platelets still contained $1-2x10^8$ leucocytes. Lopez (et al. 1990) found no such difference in AML comparing retrospectively 29 patients who received STD-transfusions with a 2 year DFS of 34% and at 4 years of 11.5%, with 28 patients who received LP transfusions containing $1-3x10^8$ leucocytes (2 year and 4 year DFS both 11.5%). Rebulla (et al. 1990) randomized AML and ALL patients to receive STD (leucocyte contamination not mentioned) and LP ($< 5x10^6$ leucocytes) red cell and platelet transfusions and found no difference in DFS, being 31% and 36% respectively at 3 years. Norol (et al. 1991) randomized

AML patients to STD red cell, random standard platelet concentrates and prophylactic granulocyte transfusions or to LP transfusions with filtered red cells and leucocyte poor apheresis platelets.

The 29 patients in the STD group and 38 patients in the LP group both had a 2 year DFS of about 42%. The total mean number of leucocytes transfused in the standard group to a patient was 3.8×10^{11} (90×10^9 lymphocytes). In the LP group these numbers were 2.9×10^{11} and 2.4×10^9 respectively. Oksanen (et al. 1993) observed in a retrospective study a longer leukaemia free survival in 65 AML patients who received filtered ($< 5 \times 10^6$ leucocytes) blood products (survival 50, 45 and 37% after 2, 3 and 4 years). The 50 patients who received STD-transfusions containing 0.5-1×10^9 leucocytes had a DFS-plateau of approximately 25% after 2, 3 and 4 years).

They showed that this improved response was largely due to the prevention of HLA antibodies enabling better platelet supportive care and thus allowing optimal chemotherapy in contrast to refractory patients. In none of the studies irradiation of blood products was mentioned although it is unusual not to irradiate granulocyte transfusions. All these studies were small and were not comparable. Among other factors, different transfusion regimens were followed. For instance the amount of leucocytes transfused in the leucocyte-poor groups in the studies of Lopez and Tucker were similar as in the standard-group in the Oksanen study. For this reasons is not possible to draw conclusions. Mature T cells from HLA-matched (marrow) donors are currently widely applied to attempt treatment of leukaemia relapse after bone marrow transplantation. In the Tucker and the Norol study the STD groups received comparable number of allogeneic lymphocytes present in single donor platelets or granulocyte transfusions respectively. Among these, HLA matched donors may have mediated a graft versus leukaemia response in individual donor-recipient combinations.

In-vitro elimination of bacterial contaminants
Freshly withdrawn blood for transfusion purposes contains in 1-4% of the units bacterial contaminants, generally from the skin at the puncture site. The great majority of such bacteriae are killed resulting in sterile cultures after a couple of days. This is often attributed to the presence of viable leucocytes and complement shortly after withdrawal. According to some investigators this phenomenon is of importance, but only for the timing of leucocyte depletion.

Concluding, leucocytes in blood transfusions have immunomodulatory effects that are beneficial in the conditioning of patients awaiting an organ transplantation and might be beneficial in immune-mediated diseases like Crohn's disease. In leukaemia patients the possibility that allogeneic leucocytes may exert a GVL is not excluded, but the concomitant induction of HLA antibodies also result in suboptimal chemotherapeutical treatment.

The immunological effects of blood transfusions are highly dependent on MHC-matching or mismatching between donor and recipient and on the presence of viable, probably non-irradiated, antigen presenting cells and immune competent T cells. Depending on the desired effect a careful selection of donor and product is necessary for individual patients with a particular disease. With this knowledge it is obsolete to rely on an effect of passenger lymphocytes in various random transfusion products to induce immunomodulation.

Positive effects of leucocyte depletion

In contrast to the limited number of available studies addressing the questions of negative effects there is abundant literature showing a beneficial effect of leucocyte-poor blood transfusions.

HLA-allo-immunization
Retrospective (Eernisse, Brand 1981) prospective (Brand et al. 1981, Murphy et al. 1986) and randomized (Schiffer et al. 1983, Murphy et al. 1986, Andreu et al. 1988, Sniecinski et al. 1988, Oksanen et al. 1991, Marwijk Kooy et al. 1991) studies demonstrated a lower rate of HLA-alloimmunization with leucocyte depleted blood products. Prevention of immunization is indicated for patients who will depend on platelet transfusions for more than a couple of weeks, organ graft recipients and life-long red cell transfusions.

CMV transmission
Prevention of transmission of primary CMV infection by blood transfusions to patients who are at risk for the development of CMV-disease was demonstrated for leukaemia patients (Graan-Hentzen et al. 1989) in allogeneic bone marrow recipients (De Witte et al. 1990) and in premature neonates (Gilbert et al. 1989). For both prevention of HLA-immunization and CMV transmission there is a critical threshold level of leucocytes between $5x10^6$-$5x10^7$ per transfusate. Leucocyte depletion below this level can reliably be obtained by validated filtration techniques.

Aggregate formation
Micro-aggregates in stored blood cause a transient reduction of circulating platelets (Bareford et al. 1987) and play a suspected, but never proven, role in post-transfusion respiratory distress and multi organ failure after massive blood transfusions. The degree of aggregate formation is dependent on the anticoagulant and red cell preservation solutions used (is enhanced in CPD blood compared to ACD) and the number of residual white cell and platelets.

In buffycoat depleted blood leaving less than $2x10^8$ leucocytes and less than $30x10^9$ platelets (for instance prepared by top and bottom buffy-coat depletion) microaggregation does not occur in stored red cells.

Assumed positive effects of leucocyte-depleted blood which need further evaluation

Perioperative infections
Reduced bacterial clearance occurs after perioperative blood transfusions (Tartter et al. 1989). Animal experiments and two randomized studies in colorectal cancer patients (Gianotti et al. 1993, Jensen et al. 1992, Houbiers et al. 1994) suggest a dose dependent deleterious effect of transfused leucocytes. It still needs further evaluation whether filtration of red cells offers advantages in this respect compared to buffycoat removal.

Endogenous viral activation
Allogeneic leucocytes induce activation and blast formation of recipient lymphocytes (Schechter et al. 1972). Upon lymphocyte activation, endogenous (latent) viruses may be induced to proliferation (Busch et al. 1992). CMV reactivation in pregnant women can be associated with congenital CMV infection of the baby. In vitro studies suggested a similar effect with HIV-infected responder lymphocytes (Busch et al. 1992). To reduce blast formation, leucocyte-depletion to a level below 5×10^6 may be necessary.

Adverse transfusion reactions
Fever, rigors and hypotension can occur after blood transfusions even after pre-transfusion filtration of products. Recent reports found an association between pretransfusion storage duration and such reactions. Measurements in stored platelet and red cell supernatants found increased levels of the pyrogenic interleukins (TNFα, IL1, IL6). Prestorage removal of leucocytes may largely prevent release of such interleukins (Muylle et al. 1993, Heddle et al. 1993).

Conclusion

Nowadays knowledge of the mechanisms of immunization and immunosuppression by allogeneic leucocytes allows no beneficial role for leucocytes in random blood transfusions. If immunosuppression is the aim, HLA-DR shared or haploidentical donors must be selected. This means there are no negative effects of leucocyte depletion of random blood transfusions except the costs.

References

Andreu G., Dewailly J., Quarte M.C., Bidet M.L. Tardivel R., Devers L., Lam Y., Soreau E., Boccaccio C., Piard N., Bidet J.M., Genetet B., Fauchet R. (1988) Prevention of HLA-immunization with leucocyte-poor packed red cells and platelet concentrates obtained by filtration, *Blood* 72: 964-969.
Bareford D., Chandler S.T., Hawker R.J. (1987) Splenic sequestration following routine blood transfusion is reduced by filtered washed blood products, *Br. J. Haematol.* 67: 177-180.

Brand A., Claas F.H.J., Voogt P.J., Wasser M.N.J.M., Eernisse J.G. (1988) Allo-immunization after leucocyte-depleted multiple random donor platelet transfusions, *Vox Sang.* 54: 160-166.

Busch M.P., Leet H., Heitman J. (1992) Allogeneic leucocytes but not therapeutic blood elements induce reactivation and dissemination of latent human immunodeficiency virus type V infection, *Blood* 8: 2128-2135.

Eernisse J.G., Brand A. (1981) Prevention of platelet refractoriness due to HLA antibodies by administration of leukocyte-poor blood components, *Exp. Hematol.* 9 (1): 77-83.

Gilbert G.L., Hayes K., Hudson I.L. et al. (1989) Prevention of transfusion-acquired cytomegalovirus infection in infants by blood filtration to remove leucocytes, *Lancet* i: 1228-1231.

Graan-Hentsen Y.C.E. de, Gratama J.W., Mudde G.C., Verdonck L.F., Houbiers J.G.A., Brand A., Sebens F.W., Van Loon A.M., The T.H., Willemze R., De Gast G.C. (1989) Prevention of primary cytomegalovirus infection in patients with hematologic malignancies by intensive white cell depletion of blood products, *Transfusion* 29: 757-760.

Gianotti L., Pyles T., Alexander J.W., Fukushima R., Babcock G.F. (1993) Identification of the blood component responsible for increased susceptibility to gut-derived infections, *Transfusion* 33: 458-465.

Heddle N.M., Klama L.N., Griffith L. Roberts R., Shukla G., Kelton J.G. (1993) A prospective study to identify the risk factor associated with acute reactions to platelet and red cell transfusions, *Transfusion* 33: 794-797.

Houbiers J.G.A. et al., Blood transfusion and colorectal cancer: Part II Postoperative infections. Submitted for publication.

Jensen L.S., Andersen A.J., Christiansen P.M., Hokland P., Juh C.O., Madson, G. Mortensen J., Moller-Sorensen C., Hokland M. (1992) Postoperative infection and natural killer cell function following blood transfusions in patients undergoing elective colorectal surgery, *Br. J. Surg.* 79: 513-516.

Lopez J., Fernandez-Villalta M.J., Gomez-Reino F., Fernandez-Ranada J.M. (1990) Absence of Graft versus Leukaemia effect of standard hemotherapy in patients with acute myeloblastic leukaemia, *Transfusion* 30: 191-192.

Marwijk-Kooy M. van, Prooyen H.C. van, Moes H.C., Bosma-Stants I., Akkerman J.W.N. (1991) The use of leukocyte-depleted platelet concentrates for the prevention of refractoriness and primary HLA alloimmunization: a prospective, randomized trial, *Blood* 77: 201-206.

Murphy M.F., Metcalfe P., Thomas H., Eve J., Ord J., Lister T.A., Waters A.H. (1986) Use of leucocyte-poor blood components and HLA-matched platelet donors to prevent HLA-alloimmunization, *Br. J. Haematol.* 62: 529-534.

Muylle L., Joos M., Wouters E., De Bock R., Peetermans M.E. (1993) Increased tumor necrosis factor α (TNFα), interleukin 1, and interleukin 6 (IL-6) levels in the plasma of stored platelet concentrates: relationship between TNFα and IL-6 levels and febrile transfusion reactions, *Transfusion* 33: 195-199.

Norol F., Parquet N., Kuentz M., Bierling P., Cordonnier C., Beaujean F., Duedari N., Vernani J.P. (1991) Absence of graft-versus-leukaemia (GVL) effect by leucocytes transfused: a prospective randomized trial in acute myeloid leukaemia (AML) patients, *Br. J. of Haemat.* 78: 591-593.

Oksanen K., Kekomäki R., Ruutu T., Koskimies S., Myllylä G. (1991) Prevention of alloimmunization in patients with acute leukaemia by use of white cell-reduced blood components - a randomized trial, *Transfusion* 31: 588-594.

Oksanen K., Elonen E. (1993) Impact of leucocyte-depleted blood components on the haemological recovery and prognosis of patients with acute myeloid leukaemia, *Br. J. Haemat.* 84: 639-647.

Opelz G., Sengar D.P.S., Terasaki P.I. (1973) Effect of blood transfusions on subsequent kidney transplants, *Transplant Proc.* 5: 253-259.

Persijn G.G., Cohen B., Lansbergen Q, Van Rood J.J. (1979) Retrospective and prospective studies on the effect of blood transfusions in renal transplantation in the Netherlands, *Transplantation* 28: 296-401.

Peters W.R., Fry R.D., Fleshman J.W., Kodner I.J. (1989) Multiple blood transfusions reduce the recurrence rate of Crohn's disease, *Dis Colon Rectum* 32: 749-753.

Post S., Kunhardt M., Sido B., Schürmann G., Herfarth C. (1992) Der Einfluss von Bluttransfusionen auf die Rezidivrate bei Morbus Crohn, *Chirurg* 63: 35-38.

Rebulla P., Pappalettera M., Barbui T., Cortelezzi A., Isacchi G., Malagnino F., Minetti B., Sirchia G. (1990) Duration of first remission in leukaemic recipients of leucocyte-poor blood components, *Br. J. Haemat.* 75: 441-442.

Schiffer C.A., Dutcher J.P., Aisner J., Hogge D., Wiernik P.H., Reilly J.P. (1983) A randomized trial of leukocyte-depleted platelet transfusion to modify alloimmunization in patients with leukemia, *Blood* 62: 815-820

Scott A.D.N., Ritchie J.K., Phillips R.K.S. (1991) Blood transfusion and recurrent Crohn's disease, *Br. J. Surg.* 78: 455-458.

Schechter G.P., Soehnlen F., McFarland W. (1972) Lymphocyte response to blood transfusion in man, *N. Engl. J. Med.* 287: 1169-1173.

Sniecinski I., O'Donnell M.R., Nowicki B., Hill L.R. (1988) Prevention of refractoriness and HLA-alloimmunization using filtered blood products, *Blood* 71: 1402-1407.

Tartter P.I. (1989) Blood transfusions and post operative infections, *Transfusion* 29: 456-459.

Tucker J., Murphy M.F., Gregory W.M., Lim J., Rohatiner A.Z.S., Waters A.H., Lister T.A. (1989) Apparent removal of graft-versus-leukaemia effect by the use of leucocyte-poor blood components in patients with acute myeloblastic leukaemia, *Br. J. Haemat.* 73: 572-581.

Williams J.G., Wong W.D., Rothenberger D.A., Goldberg S.M. (1991) Recurrence of Crohn's disease after resection, *Br. J. Surg* 78: 10-19.

Witte T. de, Schattenberg A., Dijk B.A. van, Galama J., Olthuis H., Meer J.W.W. van der, Kunst V.A.J.M. (1990) Prevention of primary cytomegalovirus infection after allogeneic bone marrow transplantation by using leucocyte-poor random blood products from cytomegalovirus unscreened bloodbank donors, *Transplantation* 50: 964-968.

Aspects of Leucocyte Depletion of Blood Components: Present Status in Japan

4 | S. Sekiguchi

Introduction

The transfusion-associated side effects: non-hemolytic febrile transfusion reactions, HLA alloimmunization, clinical refractoriness to platelets, transmission of viral disease and graft-versus-host disease, can result from leucocyte contamination in blood products. It is well recognized that leucocyte reduction in blood products reduces the side effects of blood transfusion (Sekiguchi 1993). In this article, the present status in leucocyte depletion of blood products in Japan is reviewed.

Changes in supply of whole blood and blood component products in Japan

Japan has achieved self-sufficiency in whole blood and blood component products. Figure 1 shows the changes in the number of blood donors in the last 5 years. From 1986, 400 mL donation and apheresis, in addition to the usual 200 mL donation, were introduced. The number of 200 mL donation has decreased gradually, while that of 400 mL donations has increased. The use of apheresis has increased dramatically in the past few years, accounting for 15.8% of the all donations in 1992. This tendency is continuing; in the newest report from the Japanese Red Cross Society (JRC), the percentages were 51.3% for 200 mL donation, 28.9% for 400 mL donation, and 19.8% for apheresis. In apheresis, the sum of platelet apheresis and platelet rich plasma (PRP) apheresis accounts for 50.5% of donations. As a result, though the total number of blood donors has decreased gradually, the total volume donated has increased.

The supply of blood products is shown in Table 1 and Figure 2. While the amounts of whole blood and 200 mL-derived red cell products decreased, 400 mL-derived products increased. Therefore, the total volume supplied as red cell products increased slightly. The supply of plasma products did not change. On the other hand that of platelet products increased dramatically. Though platelet products derived from whole blood decreased in absolute terms, platelet products obtained by apheresis increased rapidly. Some blood centers, including our blood center, have already changed to a system providing only apheresis-derived platelet concentrates.

Figure 1 *Annual collection of blood in Japan*

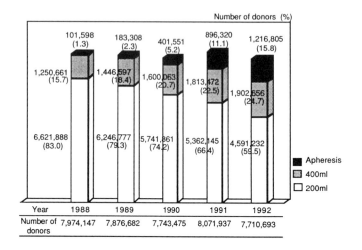

Table 1 *Distribution of blood and blood components in Japan*

	1988	1989	1990	1991	1992
Whole blood					
200 ml	1,085,246	974,350	804,011	669,171	524,935
400 ml	125,497	137,520	141,347	143,031	139,496
Red cell concentrates					
1 u*	3,448,393	3,305,043	3,050,301	2,822,885	2,621,890
2 u**	653,807	795,177	899,012	1,052,514	1,209,476
Platelet concentrates					
1 u*	2,284,232	2,167,254	1,931,110	1,582,350	1,060,085
2 u**	513,078	610,324	677,567	737,691	685,461
5 u***	32,464	49,058	78,154	170,815	289,266
10 u***	27,988	42,819	58,888	80,491	141,552
15 u***			4,358	13,373	24,544
20 u***			983	3,125	4,891
Plasma[a]					
1 u*	3,720,285	3,434,408	3,064,866	2,763,160	2,550,678
2 u**	706,996	813,716	938,178	1,051,029	1,148,946
5 u***	12,198	22,492	42,848	59,856	75,639

* derived from 200 ml whole blood donation; ** derived from 400 ml whole blood donation; *** derived from apheresis donation; [a] mainly fresh frozen plasma; u = unit.

Figure 2 *Distribution of blood and blood components in Japan*

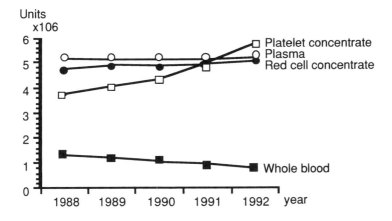

New additive solution was introduced for red cell concentrates

To prevent leucocyte-mediated side effects such as alloimmunization, leucocyte depletion and inactivation are known to be effective. There is a correlation between the number of leucocytes transfused and the occurrence of side effects, as shown in Figure 3. The concentration of contaminating leucocytes in 100 mL of various blood products prepared in our blood center is shown in Figure 4. An efficient method to reduce leucocytes in blood products is to remove buffy coat (BC) from red cell concentrates (RCC). The new additive solution, MAP (mannitol, adenin, phosphate), was introduced recently in the JRC and the MAP is added to the buffy coat-poor red cell concentrate (BPRCC). The composition of MAP is similar to the SAGM solution, but the MAP contains phosphate. Because the buffy coat is removed from the RCC, the leucocyte contamination in the BPRCC is less than that in the RCC. However, the number of leucocytes in BPRCC prepared by the top and bottom system is significantly lower than that in the BPRCC prepared by the conventional system. Though the removal rate of leucocytes is about 70-80%, only, most of the residual leucocytes are granulocytes, not lymphocytes (Nakajo et al. 1992). The number of lymphocytes was less than approximately 1x10^6 cells/bag (Table 2). The top & bottom system was recently approved by the Japanese Health and Welfare Ministry, and we have been waiting the approval by the JRC.

Figure 3 *Relationship between side effects and transfused leucocytes number*

Side effect	Major responsible cell	Leukocyte number				
		10^5	10^6	10^7	10^8	10^9
NHFTR	Granulocyte Monocyte					
HLA antibody Alloimmunization	Monocyte B lymphocyte					
HTLV-I infection	CD4+					
CMV infection	Lymphocyte Monocyte Granulocyte					
TA-GVHD	CD4+ CD8+					

■ Possible   ▨ ?   ☐ Not observed

Figure 4 *Concentration of residual leucocytes in 100 ml of RCC or PC products*

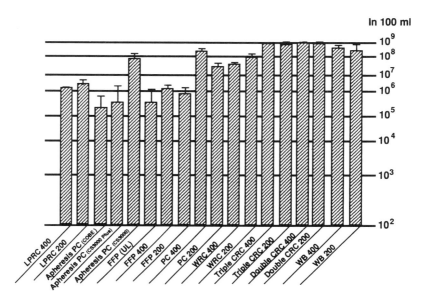

From Takahashi et al. (1993a)

Table 2 *Properties of buffy coat-poor red cell concentrates*

	Top and Bottom		Conventional	
	Separator	Optipress (BC method)	Compomat	Terumo
n	10	10	10	10
Volume (ml)	272.5 ± 13.9	248.8 ± 10.2	252.7 ± 7.2	285.0 ± 19.9
Hematocrit (%)	56.4 ± 1.9	55.0 ± 0.7	58.2 ± 1.3	61.3 ± 1.5
Leucocyte				
cells/μl (x10^3)	2.13 ± 1.21	1.89 ± 1.09	3.05 ± 1.23	4.98 ± 2.18
Removal rate (%)	78.4 ± 10.4	83.9 ± 6.6	72.0 ± 6.6	56.8 ± 11.3
Lymphocyte				
cells/μl	<18	<20	245.4 ± 106.8	687.7 ± 393.0
Removal rate (%)	>99.3	>99.6	93.9 ± 2.3	79.5 ± 13.3
Red cell				
cells/μl (x10^6)	5.98 ± 0.66	5.91 ± 0.04	6.13 ± 0.32	5.79 ± 0.04
Removal rate (%)	85.6 ± 1.8	77.2 ± 1.6	83.9 ± 1.2	91.6 ± 2.2
Platelet				
cells/μl (x10^3)	1.83 ± 0.73	2.41 ± 1.61	26.5 ± 10.3	60.4 ± 24.9
Removal rate (%)	99.5 ± 0.1	99.4 ± 0.3	94.1 ± 2.3	81.1 ± 12.2

(mean±SD)
From Nakajo et al. (1992)

Table 3 *Efficiency of 6 log filter for red cells concentrates*

	Pre-filtered leucocyte count (x10^9)	Post-filtered leucocyte count (x10^3)	Leucocyte removal rate (log)	Red cells recovery (%)	Filtration time
RZ2-1*	2.54	2.75	6.02	81.07	27'36"
	± 0.21	± 1.75	± 0.26	± 0.45	± 8'32"
RZ2-2*	2.46	4.00	6.11	81.60	34'36"
	± 0.12	± 4.95	± 0.86	±2.33	±8'03"

* tentative name (Asahi Medical)
n=6, mean±SD

Usage of leucocyte-removal filters in blood centers

The usage of leucocyte removal filters both for red cell and platelet concentrates has been increasing in Japan. However, the leucocyte-poor RCC are supplied from blood centers only when hospitals make a request to the blood center. The filters used for the leucocyte-poor RCC are Sepacell RN and Pall BPF4. Filtration of platelet products is not performed in blood centers, only at bedside. The number of leucocytes remaining in the blood products can be greatly reduced with high-efficiency leucocyte removal filters; a 6 log-reduction is achieved by the new-generation filters as shown in Table 3 (Takahashi et al. 1993a). These filters can prevent some leucocyte-mediated side effects, and the efforts to develop better filters should be continued in collaboration with filter manufacturers.

Leucocyte contamination in platelet products

The level of leucocyte contamination in the platelet concentrate by apheresis varies among apparatuses. In Figure 5, the top two panels show the appearance of conventional platelet apheresis apparatus, and the bottom two panels show those derived from improved apparatus. A reduction of contaminating leucocytes is more than 2 log in the new apparatuses. On the other hand, the products of PRP apheresis contain larger numbers of leucocytes. Table 4 shows the levels of contaminating leucocytes in the PRP products prepared by two different apparatuses. Considering that the production of PRP is high compared to that of PC apheresis, it may be necessary to combine leucocyte-depletion filter system to the apheresis systems.

Table 4 *Numbers of platelets and leucocytes in the products of platelet rich plasma*

	Haemonetics UL-PCS[1]	Autopheresis C-II[2]
Total platelets (x10^{11}/bag)	1.49 ± 0.36	2.07 ± 0.57
	(1.00 ~ 3.00)	(1.00 ~ 4.60)
Total leucocytes (x10^8/bag)	0.75 ± 0.05	2.61 ± 2.82
	(0.28 ~ 3.27)	(0.23 ~ 26.2)

[1] n=220, [2] n=221

Counting methods for the residual leucocytes in leucocyte-depleted blood products

The improvements of leucocyte removal filters and apheresis apparatus have made it difficult to count the few remaining leucocytes in blood products using automated electronic cell counters or visual counting in conventional hemocytometers. Though it is not required to report the number of contaminating leucocytes in each blood units at present, we believe it will be necessary to do so from the standpoint of quality assurance.

We have evaluated and developed three counting methods, using a Nageotte hemocytometer with a large-volume chamber (50 uL), flow cytometer and polymerase chain reaction (PCR) (Takahashi et al. 1993b). For the Nageotte chamber, we stained nuclei of leucocytes in platelet and red cell concentrate with propidium iodide (Hosoda et al. 1992).

Figure 5 *Numbers of leucocyte in apheresis-derived platelet concentrates*

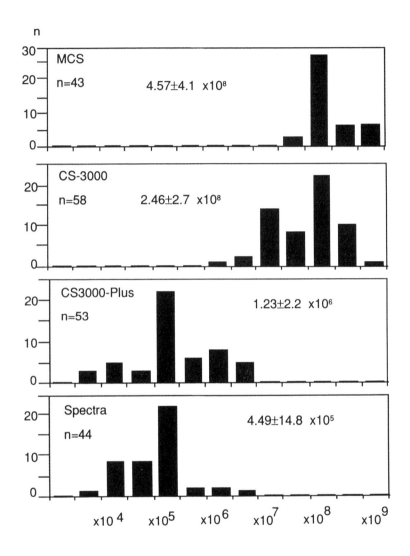

Modified from reference: Takahashi et al. (1993a)

Since we introduced the Nageotte chamber method to Japan, it has become considered as a reliable, inexpensive and easy method to count leucocytes in leucocyte-poor blood products for quality assurance. We use flow cytometric methods, with the Epics Profile II and Ortho Cytoron flow cytometers. The detection limit of the flow cytometric method is 85 cells/μL. Ten fold concentration of samples improved the detection sensitivity to 8.5 cells/mL. The leucocytes in most of the leucocyte-poor blood products can be counted by this flow cytometric method. However, it may be necessary to develop more sensitive and reliable techniques for evaluation of 6 log leucocyte removal filters.

Figure 6 *Concentration of residual leucocytes in 100 ml of PC or RCC and the sensitivity of counting methods*

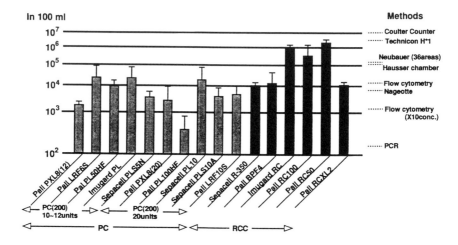

Modified from Takahashi et al. (1993)

We have applied polymerase chain reaction (PCR) to amplify the β-globin gene, which is considered as a single copy cellular gene, to detect extremely low numbers of contaminating leucocytes in filtered PC and RCC. Figure 6 summarizes the numbers of leucocytes in filtered blood products and the sensitivities of counting methods (Takahashi et al. 1993b).

Irradiation of blood products

The leucocyte depletion also contributes to prevent transfusion-transmitted virus infection, such as HTLV-I (Sekiguchi and Takahashi 1989) and CMV. However, in terms of the prevention of PT-GVHD, the removal of leucocytes may be ineffective because a very small number of leucocytes leaking into the filtrate are probably enough to trigger PT-GVHD. The incidence of PT-GVHD is quite high in Japan compared to that in other countries because of the similarity of HLA types in Japanese. Recent report of the Japanese Red Cross Society shows the incidence of PT-GVHD is 1 in about 600 cardiac surgery.

For the purpose of inactivation of leucocytes, gamma-ray or X-ray irradiation has been recommended in current practice. The JRC is planning to set up X-ray or gamma-ray irradiators in every blood center in Japan, though some of the blood centers have already installed them. The irradiation doses are recommended between 15 and 50 Gy, and the irradiated blood products are supplied only when the hospitals request them. It is necessary to await further studies to confirm whether high-efficiency leucocyte removal filters are effective in preventing PT-GVHD. On the other hand, even with gamma-ray irradiation, alloimmunization cannot be prevented. Inactivation of leucocytes by ultraviolet-B (UV-B) irradiation may prevent both GVHD and alloimmunization (Takahashi et al. 1993c). If UV-B irradiation is demonstrated to be effective in inactivating leucocytes without any deleterious side effects, such as mutation of leucocytes and/or viruses, this simple and inexpensive method will be very useful to prevent leucocyte-mediated side effects. Photoinactivation has the potential to prevent alloimmunization and GVHD in addition to the prevention of virus transmission. In our blood center, basic studies in both UV-B irradiation and photoinactivation are continuing.

Summary

The importance of leucocyte depletion of blood products has been recognized for the last few years in Japan, and blood centers show strong interests in the methods to reduce contaminating leucocytes. These efforts should be continued to abolish the leucocyte-originated side effects on blood transfusion, but with careful consideration of cost-effectiveness.

References

Hosoda M. et al. (1992) Use of the Nageotte and Hauser chambers to count residual leucocytes in leucocyte-depleted blood products, *Jpn. J. Transfus. Med.* 38: 721-727.

Nakajo S. et al. (1992) Comparison of a 'Top and Bottom' system with a conventional quadruple-bag system for blood component preparation and storage, *Jpn. J. Transfus. Med.* 38: 392-400.

Sekiguchi S. (1993) *Clinical Application of Leucocyte Depletion*, Blackwell Scientific Publications, Oxford.

Sekiguchi S. and Takahashi T.A. (1989) Leucocyte-depleted blood products and their clinical usefulness, in Brozovic B. (ed.) *The Role of Leucocyte Depletion in Blood Transfusion Practice*, Blackwell Scientific Publications, Oxford, pp. 26-34.

Takahashi T.A. et al. (1993a) Where and how the leucocytes in blood products should be depleted?, *Blood Programme* 16: 288-294.

Takahashi T.A. et al. (1993b) Comparison of highly sensitive methods used to count residual leucocytes in filtered red cell and platelet concentrates, in Sekiguchi S. (ed.) *Clinical Application of Leucocyte Depletion*, Blackwell Scientific Publications, Oxford, pp. 77-91.

Takahashi T.A. et al. (1993c) Potential involvment of free radical reactions in inactivating antigen presenting cells by ultraviolet-B irradiation, in Smit C.Th., Sibinga, Das P.C. and The T.H. (eds.) *Immunology and Blood Transfusion*, Kluwer Academic Publishers, Dordrecht, pp. 121-127.

UV Irradiation: Alternative or Supplement to Leucodepletion?

5 | G. Andreu

This work was supported by grants N° 89-CC-181 from the Ligue Nationale Française contre le Cancer (comité de Paris), N° 896897 from the Association pour la Recherche contre le Cancer and N° 90077 from the Commission de Recherche Clinique, Assistance Publique-Hôpitaux de Paris.

Introduction

Ultra Violet B (UVB) light (280-320 nm) has well identified effects on cells involved in the immune response. In vitro and animal experiments provide evidence that UVB irradiation can prevent alloimmunization against MHC class I antigens. As recent technologic improvements enable to prepare UVB irradiated platelet concentrates, the question arises of their use, in conjunction with leucocyte depletion.

We shall review the arguments that justify to investigate other means than leucodepletion for HLA alloimmunization prevention, the relevant in vitro effects of UVB irradiation, and the experimental as well as clinical data available today about the use of UVB irradiated platelets.

Analysis of HLA alloimmunization prevention with leucocyte-poor blood components

We recently analyzed (Andreu et al. 1994) the results of ten prospective randomized studies comparing the use of leuco-depleted vs standard blood components (Elghouzzi et al. 1981, Schiffer et al. 1983, Murphy et al. 1986, Sniecinski et al. 1988, Andreu et al. 1988, Rebulla et al. 1989, Van Marwijk Kooy et al. 1991, Oksanen et al. 1991, Handa et al. 1992, Andreu et al. 1993). These studies have all closely related definitions of HLA alloimmunization, i.e. a positive reaction using the microlymphocytotoxicity test with either at least 10% of a panel of 80 to 100 unselected lymphocytes or 18 to 24 cells selected according to their HLA A and B phenotype. Although all the studies show a reduction of HLA immunization frequency using leucodepleted components, only five reach statistical significance. This phenomenon is probably related to the low number of patients in the corresponding publications, except in one (Oksanen et al.), where it can be related to the very low immunization rate in the control group. Estimated Odds-ratio for the pooled studies is .31, with a 95% confidence limit of .2 to .6. Therefore, the risk to develop HLA antibodies is 3.2 times (1.7 to 5) lower with leucodepleted than with standard components.

Other aspects of HLA antibodies development that can be analyzed are their pattern - limited vs broad specificity -, and their disappearence: in comparing these characteristics in the studies where they are available (Andreu et al. 1988, Sniecinski et al. 1988, Pamphilon et al. 1989, Van Marwijk Kooy et al. 1991, Oksanen et al. 1991, Andreu et al. 1993, Waller et al. 1987, Brand et al. 1988), one can say that there is a tendency to have less antibodies with broad specificity (44% vs 60%) and more transient antibodies (29% vs 17%) in patients transfused with leucodepleted cellular blood components.

Previous stimulations with either transfusions and/or pregnancies appear as a major risk factor of HLA immunization in patients receiving leucodepleted components. Considering the ten studies as a whole, 25 out of 40 (63%) belong to that category in the immunized, vs 110 out of 259 (42%) in the non immunized patients (Chi square = 5.28, p < .025). Therefore, assuming that the use of standard blood components leads to both primary and secondary response against HLA antigens, we can conclude that leucodepleted components are more efficient to prevent primary immunization than secondary responses. This failure to prevent secondary HLA response with leucodeplcted components has been observed in other studies involving a large cohort of patients (Brand et al. 1988), or patients transfused with extremely leucodepleted components, i.e. containing less than 10^5 leucocytes per red cell or platelet concentrate (Meryman 1991), and finally in a prospective randomized study involving transfusion of female patients with a history of at least one pregnancy (Sintnicolaas et al. 1991). In the latter, the rate of immunization is equal whatever the patients receive platelet concentrates with a relatively high leucocyte content (mean = 365×10^6/unit), or leucodepleted platelet concentrates with a mean leucocyte content of 2×10^6/unit.

Therefore, despite a dramatic reduction of frequency, and less broad specific antibodies, HLA immunization remains a serious problem in 5 to 10% of multi-transfused patients. Although blood centers can provide HLA selected single donor platelet concentrates for some of these patients, any other means able to reduce this morbidity deserves to be investigated, with a special attention for procedures that could prevent secondary response.

Biological effects of UVB relevant to HLA immunization prevention

The mechanism of HLA alloantigen recognition differs from the usual way of antigen presentation as donor's antigen presenting cells (APC) can directly bind to host's CD4 cells and induce allogeneic recognition as illustrated in Figure 1. HLA immunization of recipient can be related to the fact that some endogenous peptides normally associated with HLA class II molecules of resting APC belong to HLA class I molecules (Essaket et al. 1990, Chen et al. 1990).

Figure 1 *Schematic representation of several alloreactivity pathways*

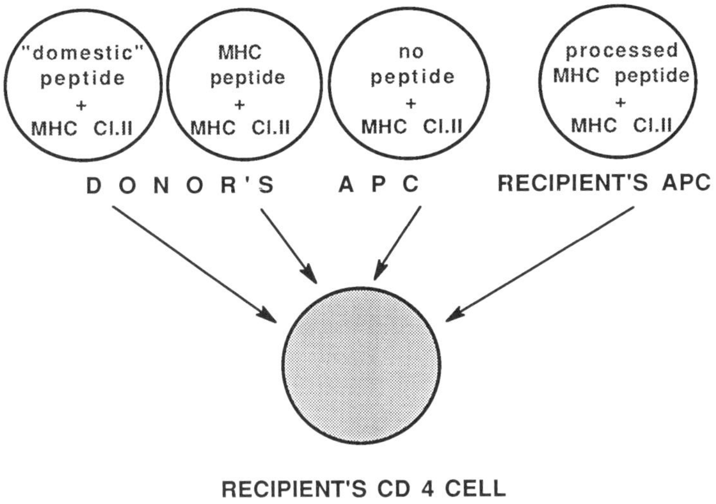

"domestic" peptide + MHC Cl.II

MHC peptide + MHC Cl.II

no peptide + MHC Cl.II

processed MHC peptide + MHC Cl.II

D O N O R ' S   A P C   RECIPIENT'S APC

RECIPIENT'S CD 4 CELL

Three cell populations can present antigen in blood:

- Dendritic cells (DC) are bone marrow-derived cells present in almost every organ, including blood: human blood MNC preparations contain from 1 to 2 % DC (Knight et al. 1986). DC have a weak phagocytic activity and a high stimulating activity in the primary MLR which functionally distinguish them from monocytes (Bjerke et al. 1985, Kuntz Crow et al. 1982).
- Monocytes, although less efficient than DC, are able of antigen presentation. Moreover, it has been shown (Kabel et al. 1989, Andreu et al. 1992) that monocytes can differentiate in vitro, and aquire all the characteristics of DC in specific culture conditions.
- B lymphocytes are also potent antigen presenting cells for T lymphocytes (Chu et al. 1984).

UVB irradiation of mononuclear cells (MNC) as a whole or purified antigen presenting cells impairs their ability to stimulate allogeneic MNC population in mixed lymphocyte reaction (MLR) (Lindahl Kiessling et al. 1971). This basic observation is the result of UVB induced modifications of antigen presentation and T cell activation.

UVB induced modifications of APC membrane molecules
MHC class II antigens are depressed after UVB irradiation, DQ and DP antigens being more sensitive than DR antigen. Such differences could be related to the different kinetics of DR, DP and DQ shedding from the cell membrane (Emerson et al. 1984). However, DR antigens on B cells are poorly sensitive to UV irradiation,

when compared to DR antigens on monocytes (Krutman et al. 1990). This apparent discrepancy cannot be related to a difference in overall protein synthesis defect which is the same for the two populations (Hertl et al. 1991) but could be related to the very active MHC class II antigen recycling by B cells (Brodsky et al. 1991).

Other proteins known to shed from cell membrane are profoundly affected by UV B irradiation, as shown in Figure 2: this is the case of ICAM 1 molecule (Hertl et al. 1991, Krutman et al. 1991) and CD 14, the lipopolysaccharide receptor on monocytes (Andreu et al. 1992). B7 (BB1) molecule, which plays a major role when combined with its ligand CD28 for T cell activation is also profoundly depressed (Young et al. 1993).

Figure 2 *Membrane proteins affected by UVB irradiation of antigen presenting cells*

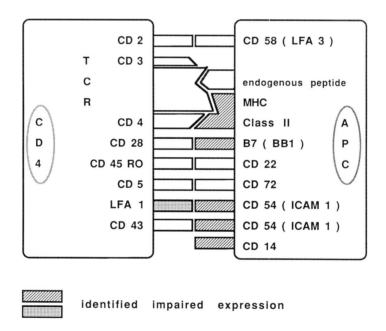

identified   impaired   expression

UVB induced modifications of APC and T cell dependent interleukins
In vitro IL-1 production by human blood monocytes stimulated with LPS is profoundly inhibited by exposure to UVB doses which inhibit their accessory cell functions (Elmets et al. 1987). Surface membrane IL-1 of macrophages is also reduced by UV B irradiation (Lange-Wantzin et al. 1987). Similar IL-1 defects have been observed after UV B irradiation of macrophages (Jackway et al. 1983), and

epidermal cells (Rich et al. 1987, Sauder et al. 1983) in mouse. However, the addition of exogenous IL-1 is not able to provide a full restoration of T cell stimulation by either allogeneic cells (Sauder et al. 1983) or antigen-pulsed macrophages (Jackway et al. 1983, Tominaga et al. 1983) and epidermal cells. This absence of complete restoration by IL-1 may be related to a defect in IL-6 production by APC, as IL-6 is an essential early signal for T cell activation by APC (Van Schnick 1990).

T cell activation is inhibited after UVB iradiation of donor's APC. IL-2 production in MLR is depressed. However, IL-2 alpha receptor (CD 25), detected early in the process of T cell activation, is produced almost normally (Mincheff et al. 1993). Small amounts of exogenous IL-2 are able to partially restore T cell proliferation in MLR (Tominaga et al. 1983), restoration being more efficient when IL-2 is added at 8 or 16 hours of culture vs 2 hours (Mincheff et al. 1993, Young et al. 1993).

All these modifications of T cell activation fit with the following sequence of events after UVB irradiation of donor's APC:

- contact between APC and resting alloreactive CD4 cell is almost normal, leading to the production of CD 25 receptor on cell membrane.
- However, APC are not able to produce a costimulatory signal necessary for full T cell activation. In normal conditions, the contact between B7 receptor on APC and its ligand CD28 on CD4 cells leads to autocrine IL-2 production, which initiates T cell proliferation. The lack of sufficient B7 receptors after UVB irradiation (Young et al. 1993) accounts for the absence of T cell proliferation.

Other cell membrane modifications of T cell subpopulations following UVB irradiation have been described, as a depression of adhesion molecule LFA 1 (Deeg et al. 1987), or cytotoxicity alteration (Kobata et al. 1993). However, these events are not directly relevant to the onset of alloimmunization.

UVB induction of T suppressor cell population
The lack of a costimulatory signal for T cell activation does not imply a simple absence of alloreactivity, but can lead to a state of tolerance mediated by the generation of T suppressor cells. The production of a T suppressor population following UVB irradiation has been demonstrated in various experimental conditions (Greene et al. 1979, Oluwole et al. 1989, Lau et al. 1983, Oluwole et al. 1985). The mechanism of UVB irradiated donor specific transfusions effect in rat heart allograft has been approached: purified 0x8+ lymphocytes (the equivalent of CD8+ in human) from Lewis animals permanently tolerant to ACI transplanted heart after UVB irradiated donor specific transfusions induce a significant donor specific enhancement of graft survival in naive syngeneic hosts (Oluwole et al. 1989). Therefore, UVB irradiated donor specific transfusions effect is at least in part related to the development of a specific suppressive lymphocyte population in the future transplant recipient.

Effect of UVB on immune secondary response in vitro

We conducted the following in vitro experiments relevant to the prevention of alloimmunization (Andreu et al. 1992): MNC were primed by culture for 10 days in culture flasks with mitomycin-treated stimulating allogeneic cells, and boosted with either untreated or UVB irradiated (0.3 J/cm2) stimulating cells. Secondary response was evaluated by ^{3}H-thymidine incorporation after 48 additional hours of culture. The results show unequivocally that UVB irradiation completely inhibits secondary response. We can conclude that UVB impairs allogeneic antigen presentation, not only to naive T cells, but also to already primed cells.

Conversely, when MNC are primed with UVB irradiated dendritic cells, and boosted with untreated irradiated stimulating cells, the secondary response is delayed and weaker than the proliferation of the same cells primed with untreated dendritic cells. However, this experiment is difficult to interpret, as the generation of cytotxic T cells after secondary culture was not checked. When, in the same experiment scheme, primary culture has been supplemented by exogenous IL-2, primary and secondary proliferations have a normal pattern (Young et al. 1993).

Prevention of transfusion induced MHC class I alloimmunization with UVB irradiation

Animal experiments

Transfusion of UV-C irradiated diluted blood in dogs prevents alloimmunization against class I MHC antigens (Slichter et al. 1987): in experimental conditions consisting of 8 weekly single donor random transfusions, where more than 85% of dogs (18/21) were immunized against allogeneic class I MHC antigens, UV-C irradiation of the transfused products could reduce the immunization rate to less than 10% (1/12). Moreover, once transfused for 8 weeks with UV-C irradiated components, a high proportion of dogs (8/11) remains unimmunized, even if submitted to an intensive transfusion regimen with non UV-C irradiated components from the same donor, known to be extremely immunogenic in previously untransfused dogs. These 8 non refractory recipients were transfused with components from two or three other random donors until immunization occurred or a maximum of 8 transfusions of each of these new donors had been given. 10 out of 23 donors could not elicit alloimmunization. Finally, 6 of the nonimmunized recipients were transfused with platelets from their original donor and immunization occurred in 2. It is important to note that these 2 immunizations appeared more than 3 months after the end of the series of 8 transfusions.

In a mouse model of MHC class I alloimmunization where after two transfusions 100% of recipients of standard platelet concentrates were immunized, leucocyte depletion and UVB irradiation were compared (Kao 1992): leucocyte depletion could prevent immunization in 50%, and UVB in 100% of the animals. After four transfusions, all recipients of leucocyte-depleted platelet concentrates were immunized, while 60% of recipients of UVB irradiated platelet concentrates were not. Moreover, post-transfusion platelet recovery was in the normal range in all recipients of UVB irradiated, and frankly abnormal in 4 out of 5 recipients of leucocyte-depleted platelet concentrates. Finally, when non immunized mice previously transfused with UVB irradiated products were challenged with standard platelet concentrates, they did develop antibodies which remained with significantly lower titre than those of controls.

Clinical trials using UVB irradiated platelets
In the first trial reported newly diagnosed patients with malignancy and anticipated long term platelet transfusion needs were randomized to receive either untreated or UVB irradiated (8-15 J/cm2) PC (Buchholz et al. 1990). In the two groups, red cell transfusion was carried on with leucodepleted products using the Sepacell R500 (Asahi, Japan) filter. The 17 patients in the control group and the 22 patients receiving UVB irradiated PC did not differ in regard to age, sex ratio, time in study and number of RCC and PC transfusion. HLA immunization was evaluated as the mean percentage of panel lymphocytotoxicity, which was 4.4% in the UVB group and 30.5% in the control group (p = 0.007). Refractoriness to platelet transfusions was observed in 6 patients in each group. However, refractoriness could be clearly related to HLA alloimmunization in 5 out of 6 patients in the control group and in 2 out of 6 patients in the UV group. These two patients were female (previous pregnancies are not mentioned).

These results should be interpreted having in mind that 10 to 15% of the RCC filtrated with the Sepacell R500 filter contain more than 5×10^6 residual leucocytes (Masse et al. 1991). Therefore, these non UVB treated leucocytes present in red cell products could be responsible of HLA alloimmunization.

We conducted a multicenter study in France (Andreu et al. 1993). All the patients received leucocyte-depleted red cell concentrates, and the control counts showed that more than 98% of RCC contained less than 10^6 residual leucocytes. Patients were randomized in three groups: in the control group, patients received platelet concentrates containing a median of 200×10^6 leucocytes; in the UVB group, platelet concentrates with a similar leucocyte content were irradiated in controlled conditions with the energy of 0.5 J/cm2; and the third group was transfused with leucocyte-depleted platelet concentrates, containing a median of 0.37×10^6 leucocytes. 7 patients among 22 (31.8%) in the control group developed HLA antibodies, 4 being with a broad specificity. In contrast, 3 out of 26 (11.5%) and 3 out of 28 (10.7%) were HLA immunized in the leucocyte-poor and UV-B group respectively (differences not statistically significant when the leucocyte-poor group and the UV-B group are considered separately against control). Analysis of patients' history of transfusions and pregnancies lead to the conclusion that primary response occurred in 3 out of 7 in the control group, none out of 3 in the leucocyte-depleted and 2 out of 3 in the UVB group.

Conclusion

The use of leucocyte-depleted cellular components reduces the onset of HLA alloimmunization quantitatively and qualitatively. The remaining immunization rate leads to difficulties of platelet transfusion support in 5 to 10% of multitransfused patients. UVB irradiation, although usable only for platelet concentrates, deserves to be investigated as a means to reduce this morbidity, for at least two reasons:

- filtration technology available today, even highly sophisticated, does not ensure a complete elimination of leucocytes from cellular blood components.
- UVB mechanism of action of is completely different from that of leucocyte depletion; we can expect from in vitro experiments that it could be efficient on secondary responses, which leucodepletion fails to prevent.

UVB trials already performed showed that this treatment, when properly done, does not impair post transfusion platelet recovery. However, apart from the effect on HLA alloimmunization prevention, careful clinical record of all patients transfused in this way must be kept, as we have to investigate the possible deleterious effects of the UVB-induced immunomodulation.

Apart from the prevention of HLA alloimmunization, leucocyte depletion of cellular components has been shown useful in many ways in transfusion practice to reduce the frequency of febrile non hemolytic transfusion reactions (Lieden et al. 1982, Sirchia et al. 1986); to improve the storage conditions of either red cell concentrates (RCC) and platelet concentrates (PC), at least when performed early after component preparation (Angué et al. 1989); to reduce the probability of some bacterial growth, when performed in the process of component preparation (Högman et al. 1992, Gong et al. 1993); and to reduce the transmission of viruses exclusively present in leucocytes in blood, such as CMV (Andreu 1991) or HTLV I/II (Kobayashi et al. 1993). Therefore, UVB irradiation of platelet concentrates must be considered in the future only if its action is synergistic with leucocyte depletion. This analysis led us to carry on a new trial comparing a control group of patients receiving leucocyte-poor platelet concentrates with a group receiving leucocyte-poor and UV-B irradiated platelet concentrates.

References

Aberer W.G., Leibl H. (1987) Effect of UV B radiation on the biosynthesis of HLA DR antigens, *Arch. Dermatol Res* 279: 321-326.

Andreu G., Dewailly J., Leberre C., Quarre M.C., Bidet M.L., Tardivel R., Devers L., Lam Y., Soreau E., Boccaccio C., Piard N., Bidet J.M., Genetet B., Fauchet R. (1988) Prevention of HLA immunization with leucocyte-poor packed red cells and platelet concentrates obtained by filtration, *Blood* 72 (3): 964-969.

Andreu G. (1991) Role of leukocyte depletion in the preservation of transfusion - induced cytomegalovirus infection, *Seminars in Hematology* 28 (3, Suppl. 5): 26-31.

Andreu G., Perrot J.Y., Pirenne F., Boccaccio C. (1992) The effect of UVB light on antigen presenting cells (APC). Implications for transfusion-induced sensitization, *Seminars in Hematology* 29: 122-131.

Andreu G., Boccaccio C., Klaren J., Lecrubier Ch., Pirenne F., Garcia I., Baudard M., Devers L., Fournel J.J. (1992) The role of UV radiation in the prevention of HLA alloimmunization, *Transfusion Medicine Reviews* 6: 212-224.

Andreu G., Norol F., Schooneman F., Coffe C., Pouthier F., Soulier J., Traineau R., Klaren J. (1993) Prevention of HLA alloimmunization using UV-B irradiated platelet concentrates (PC): results of a prospective randomized study AABB 46th annual meeting, Miami beach, October 23-28.

Angué M., Chatelain P., Fiabane S. et al. (1989) Viabilité des globules rouges humains conservés pendant 35 jours après déplétion en leucocytes, *Rev. Fr. Transf. Hémobiol.* 32: 27-36.

Bjercke S., Gaudenack G. (1985) Dendritic cells and monocytes as accessory cells in T cell responses in man II: function as antigen presenting cells, *Scand. J. Immunol.* 21: 501-508.

Brand A., Claas F.H.J., Voogt P.J., Wasser N.M.J.M., Eernisse J.G. (1988) Alloimmunization after leukocyte-depleted multiple random donor platelet transfusions, *Vox Sang.* 54: 160-166.

Brodsky F.M., Guagliardi L.E. (1991) The cell biology of antigen processing and presentation, *Ann. Rev. Immunol.* 9: 707-744.

Buchholz D.H., Anderson J., Lin A., Hedberg S., Seagraves P., Ellis G., Aster R., Kagen L., Snyder E., Napychank P., Greenwalt T., Manitove J. (1990) Preliminary observations on UVB irradiated platelet concentrates and patient alloimmunization. Presented at the AABB/ISBT meeting, Los Angeles, November 1990.

Chen B.P., Madrigal A., Parham P. (1990) Cytotoxic T cell recognition of an endogenous class I HLA peptide presented by class II HLA molecule, *J. Exp. Med.* 172: 779-788.

Chu E., Umetsu D., Lareau M., Schneeberger E., Geha R.A. (1984) Analysis of antigen uptake and presentation by Epstein-Barr virus transformed human lymphoblastoid B cells, *Eur. J. Immunol.* 14: 291-298.

Deeg H.J., Aprile J., Severns E., Rajantie J., Schmidt E., Raff R.F., Green K.E., Storb R. (1987) Phenotypic and functional alterations of recipient lymphocytes after transfusion of UV irradiated and normal blood. Implications for marrow transplantation, *Transplant Proc.* 19: 2709.

Deeg H.J., Sigaroudinia M. (1990) Ultraviolet B-induced loss of HLA class II antigen expression on lymphocytes in dose, time and locus dependent, *Exp. Hematol.* 18: 916-919.

Elghouzzi M.H., Vedrenne J.B., Jullien A.M., Delcey D., Nadal M., Habibi B. (1981) Etude technique immunologique et clinique des performances de filtration du sang à l'aide de l'appareil Erypur, *Rev. Fr. Transfus. Immunohématol.* 24 (6): 579-595.

Elmets C.A., Larson K., Urda G.A., Schacter B. (1987) Inhibition of post binding target cell lysis and of lymphokine-induced enhancement of human natural killer cell activity by in vitro exposure to ultraviolet B radiation, *Cell. Immunol.* 104: 47-58.

Emerson S.G., Pretell J., Cone R.E. (1984) Physical and pharmacologic inhibition of the shedding of Ia antigens, *Exp. Clin. Immunogenet.* 1: 9.

Essaket S., Fabron J., De Preval C., Thomsen M. (1990) Corecognition of of HLA-A1 and HLA-DPw3 by a human CD4+ alloreactive T lymphocyte clone, *J. Exp. Med.* 172: 387-390.

Gong J., Högman C.F., Hambraeus A., Johansson C.S., Eriksson L. (1993) Transfusion-transmitted Yersinia Enterocolitica infection: protection through buffy-coat removal and failure of the bacteria to grow in platelet rich or platelet poor plasma, *Vox Sang.* 65: 42-46.

Greene M.I., Sy M.S., Kripke M., Benacerraf B. (1979) Impairment of antigen - presenting cell function by ultra-violet irradiation, *P.N.A.S.* 76 (2): 6591-6595.

Handa M., Ikeda Y., Kurata Y., Tsubaki K., Horiuchi A., Furihata K., Kimura Y., Toyama K., Takamoto S., Tsukimoto I., Yoshida H., AsaiI T., Itoh T., Baba M., Niikura H., Terada H., Miyamoto M., Sasagawa S., Sekiguchi S., Ninomiya K., Masuda M., Mizogushi H., Takahashi M., Shimizu M. (1992) Efficacy of leukocyte-depleted platelet concentrates for prevention of HLA alloimmunization in patients with frequent platelet transfusions: a prospective multiinstitutional study using a polyester platelet filter, *Jpn J. Clin. Hematol.* 33 (4): 451-460.

Hertl M., Kaplan D.R., Fayen J.D., Panuska J.R., Ellner J.J., Elmets C.A. (1991) The accessory function of B lymphocytes is resistant to the adverse effects of UV radiation, *Eur. J. Immunol.* 21: 291-297.

Högman C.F., Gong J., Eriksson L., Hambraeus A., Johansson C.S. (1992) The role of white cells in the transmission of Yersinia Enterocolitica in blood components, *Transfusion* 32: 673-676.

Jackway J.P., Shevach E.M. (1983) Stimulation of T-cell activation by UV-treated, antigen-pulsed macrophages. Evidence for a requirement for antigen processing and interleukin -1 secretion, *Cell. Immunol.* 80: 151-162.

Kabel P.J., De Haan-Meulman M., Woorbij A.M., Kleingeld M., Knol E.F., Drexhage H.A. (1989) Accessory cells with a morphology and marker pattern of dendritic cells can be obtained from elutriator-purified blood monocyte fractions. An enhancing effect of metrizamide in this differentiation, *Immunobiol.* 179: 395-411.

Kao K.J. (1992) Effects of leukocyte depletion and UVB irradiation on alloantigenicity of major histocompatibility complex antigens in platelet concentrates: a comparative study, *Blood* 80: 2931-2937.

Knight S.C., Farrent J., Bryhan A., Edwards A.J., Burman S., Lever A., Clarcke J., Webster A.D.B. (1986) Non adherent, low density cells from human peripheral blood contain dendritic cells, both with veiled morphology, *Immunology* 57: 595-603.

Kobata T., Ikeda H., Ohnishi Y., Urushibara N., Takahashi T., Sekigushi S. (1993) UV irradiation can induce in vitro clonal anergy in alloreactive cytotoxic T lymphocytes, *Blood* 82: 176-181.

Kobata T., Ikeda H., Ohnishi Y., Urushibara N., Nakata S.O., Takahashi T., Sekiguchi S. (1993) Ultraviolet irradiation inhibits killer-target cell interaction, *Vox Sang.* 65: 25-31.

Kobayashi M., Yano M., Kwon K.W., Takahashi T.A., Ikeda H., Sekiguchi S. (1993) Leukocyte depletion of HTLV I carrier red cell concentrates by filters, in: Sekuguchi S. (ed.) *Cinical Application of Leukocyte Depletion*, Blackwell Scientific Publications.

Krutman J., Khan I.U., Wallis R.S., Zhang F., Rich E.A., Ellner J.J., Elmets C.A. (1990) Cell membrane is a major locus for ultraviolet B induced alterations in accessory cells, *J. Clin. Invest.* 85: 1529-1536.

Kuntz Crow M., Kunkel H.G. (1982) Human dendritic cells: major stimulators of the autologous and allogeneic mixed leukocyte reactions, *Clin. Exp. Immunol.* 49: 338-346.

Lange-Wantzin G., Rothlein R., Kahn J., Faanes R.B. (1987) Effect of UV irradiation on membrane IL-1 by rat macrophages, *J. Immunol.* 138: 3803-3807.

Lau H., Reemtsma K., Hardy M.A. (1983) Pancreatic islet allograft prolongation by donor specific blood transfusions treated with ultraviolet irradiation, *Science* 221: 754.

Lieden G., Hildén J.O. (1982) Febrile transfusion reactions reduced by use of buffy-coat-poor erythrocytes concentrates, *Vox Sang.* 43: 263-265.

Lindahl-kiessling K., Safwenberg J. (1971) Inability of UV-irradiated lymphocytes to stimulate allogeneic cells in mixed lymphocyte culture, *Int. Arch. Allergy* 41: 670-678.

Masse M., Andreu G., Angué M., Babault C., Beaujean F., Bidet M.L., Boudart D., Calot J.P., Cotte C., Follea G., Gerota J., Hau F., Hurel C., Legrand E., Marchesseau B., Nasr O., Robert F., Royer D., Schoneman F., Tardivel R., Vidal Obert M. (1991) A multi-centre study on the efficiency of leukocyte depletion by filtration of red cells, *Transfusion* 31 (9): 792-797.

Meryman H.T. (1991) A clinical trial of leukocyte-depleted platelet transfusions in bone marrow transplanted patients. 3rd regional ISBT meeting, Prague, October 13, 1991.

Mincheff M.S., Meryman H.T., Kapoor V., Alsop P., Wötzel M.M. (1993) Blood transfusion and immunomodulation: a possible mechanism, *Vox Sang.* 65: 18-24.

Murphy M.F., Metcalfe P., Thomas H., Eve J., Ord J., Lister T.A., Waters A.H. (1986) Use of leucocyte-poor blood components and HLA-matched-platelet donors to prevent HLA allo-immunization, *Br. J. Haematol.* 62: 529-534.

Oksanen K., Kekomäki R., Ruutu T., Koskimies S., Myllylä G. (1991) Prevention of alloim-munization in patients with acute leukemia by use of leukocyte-depleted blood compo-nents - a randomized trial, *Transfusion* 31: 588-594.

Oluwole S.F., Reemtsma K., Hardy M. (1989) Characteristics and function of suppressor T lymphocytes in immunologically unresponsive rats following pretreatment with UVB irradiated donor leukocytes and peritransplant cyclosporine, *Transplantation* 47: 1001-1007.

Oluwole S.F., Iga C., Lau H., Hardy M. (1985) Prolongation of rat heart allograft by donor specific blood transfusion treated with ultraviolet irradiation, *Heart Transplant.* 4: 385.

Pamphilon D.H., Farrell D.H., Donaldson C., Raymond P.A., Brady C.A., Bradley B.A. (1989) Development of lymphocytotoxic and platelet reactive antibodies: a prospective study in patients with acute leukemia, *Vox Sang.* 57: 177-181.

Rebulla P., Andreis C., Barbui T., Bellavita P., Boeri M., Carminati V., Greppi N., Isacchi G., Lecchi L., Maiolo A.T., Malagnino F., Mandelli F., Minetti B., Quarti C., Riccardi D., Scudeller G., Sirchia G. (1989) A clinical trial on the efficacy of leukocyte-depleted blood components in preventing refractoriness to random platelet support: an interim report, in: Barbui, T., Falanga A., Minetti B., Gorini S., Tognoni G., Donati M.D. (eds.) *Infection and Haemorrhage in Acute Leukemia*, John Libbey Eurotext, Paris, pp 89-100.

Rich E.A., Elmets C.A., Fujirawa H., Wallis R.S., Ellner J.J. (1987) Deleterious effect of ultra-violet-B radiation on accessory function of human adherent MNC. *Clin. Exp. Immunol.* 70: 116-126.

Sauder D.N., Noonan F.P., De Fabo E.C., Katz S.I. (1983) Ultraviolet radiation inhibits allo-antigen presentation by epidermal cells: partial reversal by the soluble epidermal cell prod-uct, epidermal cell-derived thymocyte-activating factor (ETAF), *J. Invest. Dermatol.* 80: 485-489.

Schiffer C.A., Dutcher J.P., Aisner J., Hogge D., Wiernik P.H., Reilly J.P. (1983) A randomized trial of leukocyte-depleted platelet transfusion to modify alloimmunisation in patients with leukemia, *Blood* 62 (4): 815-820.

Sintnicolaas K., Van Prooijen H.C., Van Marwijk Kooy M., Van Dijk B.A., Van Putten W.L.J., Brand A. (1991) Leukocyte depletion of random single donor platelet transfusions for the prevention of secondary HLA alloimmunization, European Society for Hemapheresis 8th meeting, Würsburg, September 11-14, 1991.

Sirchia G., Rebulla P., Mascaretti L. et al. (1986) The clinical importance of leukocyte depletion in regular erythrocyte transfusions, *Vox Sang.* 51: 2-8.

Slichter S.J., Deeg H.J., Kennedy M. (1987) Prevention of platelet alloimmunization in dogs with systemic cyclosporine and by UV-irradiation or cyclosporine-loading of donor platelets, *Blood* 69 (2): 414-418.

Sniecincki I., O'Donnell M.R., Nowicki I.B., Hill L.R. (1988) Prevention of refractoriness and HLA allo immunization using filtered blood products, *Blood* 71 (5): 1402-1407.

Tominaga A., Lefort S., Michel S.B., Danbrawkas J.T., Granstein R., Lowy A., Benacerraf B., Greene M.I. (1983) Molecular signals in antigen presentation I: effects of interleukin 1 and 2 on radiation treated antigen presenting cells in vivo and in vitro, *Clin. Immunol. Immuno-path* 29: 282.

Van Marwijk Kooy M., Van Prooijen H.C., Moes M. (1991) Use of leukocyte-depleted platelet concentrates for the prevention of refractoriness and primary HLA alloimmunization: a prospective, randomized trial, *Blood* 77: 201-205.

Van Schnick (1990) Interleukin-6: an overview, *Ann. Rev. Immunol.* 8: 253-278.

Waller C., Urlacher A., Fischbach M., Tongio M.M., Noss P., Weill D., Geissert J., Mayer S. (1987) Immunisations HLA consécutives à des transfusions de sang déleucocyté, *Rev. Fr. Transfusion et Immunohématologie* 30 (3): 155-167.

Young J.W., Baggeers J., Soergel S.A. (1993) High dose UV-B radiation alters human dendritic cell costimulatory activity but does not allow dendritic cells to tolerize T lymphocytes to alloantigen in vitro, *Blood* 81: 2987-2997.

Mononuclear Cell Microchimerism and the Immunomodulatory Effect of Transfusion

6 | W.H. Dzik

The ability to exchange human tissue has long been a fascination of medicine and our century has witnessed progress in the biology of tissue transfer which would not have been imagined in times past. The transfusion of allogeneic human blood is the most commonplace example of human tissue transfer and it is not surprising that increased insight into the human immune system should parallel new understanding of the subtle ways in which allogeneic transfusion affects the immune system of the recipient. Although the more obvious alloimmunization effects of transfusion were the first to be recognized, a subtle immunosuppressive effect has been suspected for several decades. The clinical expression of this suspected effect has not been conclusively proven, but transfusion has been linked to the development of immunological tolerance to solid organ allografts, to increased susceptibility to viral or bacterial infection, and to a breakdown in immune surveillance against tumors (Blumberg and Heal 1994, Brunson and Alexander 1990, Triulzi et al. 1990, Van Aken 1989).

Several hypotheses have been put forward to explain the transfusion effect. Early proposed mechanisms included patient selection bias, clonal deletion of primed cells by immunosuppressive drugs (Terasaki 1984), the development of antiidiotype antibodies (Reed et al. 1987) or suppressor T cells (Leivestad and Thorsby 1984, Hutchinson 1986). Subsequent proposed mechanisms have included passive infusion of immune complexes or soluble antigens, transfusion of antibody coated cells (Susal et al. 1990), recipient exposure to plasma factors that release prostaglandin E_2 (Shelby et al. 1987, Ross et al. 1990) or immunosuppression from either plasticizers or cellular debris (Brunson and Alexander 1990). In this chapter I discuss a current hypothesis that leucocyte microchimerism resulting from blood transfusion is one of the mechanisms underlying the immunosuppressive effect of blood transfusion. The hypothesis is stated as follows: Among donor-recipient pairs who are sufficiently HLA similar, transient leucocyte microchimerism develops and extends the limits of recipient active tolerance or anergy. Critical features of this hypothesis are: 1) The transfusion effect depends on recipient exposure to viable allogeneic donor mononuclear cells; 2) the HLA relationship between the donor and recipient dictates the occurrence of the effect; 3) mononuclear cells are able to persist in low levels in the recipient (microchimerism); and 4) the persistence of donor cells is able to extend the limits of tolerance or anergy of the recipient. Each of these will be discussed in the context of blood transfusion.

The transfusion effect depends upon recipient exposure to allogeneic mononuclear cells

A large amount of experimental evidence suggests that the transfusion effect depends upon recipient exposure to allogeneic donor leucocytes (Brunson and Alexander 1990, Meryman 1989). Most early studies of pretransplant transfusion found that component preparations such as frozen-deglycerolized Red Cells or stored Red Cell Concentrates were less effective than fresh transfusions at mediating the effect. Moreover, in the study by Okazaki et al. (1985) the pretransplant transfusion effect was produced by transfusion of buffy coat cells. Subsequent studies which observed higher infection rates among recipients of allogeneic versus autologous transfusions suggested that factors such as blood additives or plasticizers which would be common to both preparations were unlikely to account for the transfusion effect. Recently, experimental studies of tumor growth in animals (Blajchman et al. 1993) and clinical trials examining postoperative infection in humans (Jensen et al. 1992) have observed that the transfusion effect depends upon recipient exposure to allogeneic leucocytes and that leucocyte depletion appears to eliminate the effect. Although there is no consensus on which lymphocyte subsets may be responsible for the transfusion effect, most studies have implicated donor T cells or donor stem cells. The term mononuclear cells is meant to refer to lymphocytes, monocytes, and stem cells.

The transfusion effect may depend on the HLA relationship between donor and recipient

Clinical studies of tumor recurrence or postoperative infection have not adequately considered that the HLA relationship between the blood donor and the transfusion recipient may be critically important for the development of transfusion-induced immunomodulation. As a result the transfusion effect may not be equally expressed in all individuals transfused with leucocyte containing blood components. For example, during the period in which pretransplant blood transfusions were given to improve renal allograft survival, it was found that random transfusions did not always produce a tolerogenic effect. Donor-specific transfusions (DSTs) were found to be more effective than random transfusions. Although many explanations are possible for the improved response following DSTs, these transfusions represented instances in which the donor and recipient were related and therefore frequently shared at least one HLA haplotype and in which the recipient was given mild immunosuppression at the time of transfusion. Such conditions may promote mononuclear cell microchimerism.

It is well known that cells in mixed lymphocyte culture react poorly with allogeneic cells that are identical at Class II antigens even if different at Class I antigens. This suggests that when transfusions are given from a donor who matches the recipient at Class II antigens, the donor cells may not elicit a strong allotransplantation response *in vivo* and thereby have an opportunity for temporary engraftment. Animal and clinical studies have also suggested that the transfusion effect occurs when the donor-recipient pair are matched at HLA-DR antigens. Quigley et al. used a rat transfusion model to study reactivity of animals transfused with blood from donors who were completely matched, partially matched, or unmatched for histocompatibility antigens (Quigley et al. 1989). The *in vitro* mixed lymphocyte response to stimulation by cells obtained from the original blood donor strain was significantly less if the responder had been transfused with matched or partially matched transfusions compared with unmatched transfusions. Similar results were obtained in humans by Leivestad in a study of HLA haploidentical DSTs (Leivestad and Thorsby 1984). Lagaaij et al. transfused 62 patients awaiting renal or cardiac transplants with a single unit of blood from *unrelated* donors who were selected for partial HLA matching with the recipient (Lagaaij et al. 1989). Among blood donor and recipient pairs who shared one HLA-DR antigen, five year graft survival (81%) was significantly higher than that observed in the absence of HLA-DR matching (57%). More recently, van Twuyer et al studied 23 patients given deliberate transfusions prior to renal transplant (Van Twuyer et al. 1991). They determined the frequency of cytotoxic T-cell precursors specific for donor cells before and after transfusion. T-cell nonresponsiveness against donor cells developed in 10 of 23 patients after transfusion. Nonresponsiveness developed only if the donor and the recipient were a one HLA-haplotype match or if they shared one HLA-B plus one HLA-DR antigen. In fact, there is a suggestion from one retrospective study that renal allograft survival following one haplotype matched DSTs was better if the donor and recipient were discordant at the other Class II antigen compared with donor-recipient pairs who matched at both Class II antigens (Lazda et al. 1990).

An obvious objection to the requirement for some degree of donor-recipient HLA similarity in the development of the transfusion effect is the infrequency with which donor-recipient transfusion pairs would be HLA matched. HLA matching based on private allele assignments has been the traditional manner of studying the role of HLA matching on the survival of transplanted bone marrow and solid organ grafts. In the setting of random transfusions, HLA matching at private allele assignments would not be expected to occur with sufficient frequency to explain the observed incidence of mild immunosuppression after transfusion. However, previous studies (cited above) suggest that the induction of nonresponsiveness may only depend upon matching at Class II loci. Moreover, the context of donor-recipient HLA similarity can be broadened by consideration of HLA cross-reactive groups, HLA public antigens, non-inherited maternal antigens, and non-serologically defined antigens.

Serologically cross-reactive antigens and public antigens represent groupings of HLA private antigen specificities which may be immunologically similar in *in vivo* situations. For example, in the setting of platelet alloimmunization to HLA antigens, platelets donated by individuals who match the recipient at public antigens (or in some cases at cross reactive antigens) can result in successful increments despite not matching the recipient at private HLA antigens. Noninherited maternal antigens refer to HLA antigens present on the maternal chromosome that was not inherited by the child. Because the child was exposed to these antigens while in utero and because the neonatal immune system is particularly prone to the development of tolerance, there is the suggestion that individuals are more tolerant to their noninherited maternal antigens (Claas et al. 1988). The van Rood group demonstrated that cytotoxic T cell precursors in children were absent or significantly diminished against noninherited maternal antigens compared with noninherited paternal antigens (Van Rood and Claas 1990). In addition, suppressed mixed lymphocyte reactions to donor cells were found after transfusion when the donor expressed noninherited maternal antigens of the recipient (Bean et al. 1990).

Finally, it should be noted that the bulk of our understanding of HLA antigens derives from antigenic specificities as determined by alloantibodies. Other cell surface structures on the HLA molecule may be more readily recognized as alloepitopes by recipient T cells. These nonserologically defined antigens may play an important role in cellular allorecognition and may open opportunities for HLA similarity between blood donors and recipients which would not be appreciated from a consideration of HLA antigens as currently defined.

Microchimerism after transfusion: along the spectrum from alloimmunization to graft vs host disease

The development of mononuclear cell microchimerism after transfusion is likely to depend not only on recipient exposure to viable allogeneic donor leucocytes but also on the extent of HLA similarity between donor and recipient - two conditions that may also be of prime importance for the development of the transfusion effect. Because HLA is the dominant transplantation alloantigen system and because donor mononuclear cells strongly express HLA antigens, it is logical to expect that the HLA similarity of the donor-recipient pair would play a critical role in the survival of transfused allogeneic donor mononuclear cells. Microchimerism can be seen as occupying a middle position on a spectrum between alloimmunization and graft-vs-host disease (see Figure 1). Among immunologically normal and responsive recipients who are exposed to completely HLA-dissimilar allogeneic leucocytes, alloimmunization is to be expected. At the other extreme are nonirradiated transfusions containing viable lymphocytes given either to recipients with severe immunodeficiency or donated from HLA homozygous donors who share one haplotype with the recipient. Such circumstances allow for engraftment, rapid clonal expansion of the donor cells, and graft versus host disease. Between these extremes may be circumstances in which donor cells are neither quickly eliminated from the host nor are allowed unchecked clonal expansion. Instead, a balanced state of microchimerism may ensue.

In addition to HLA similarity between donor and recipient, other factors may allow donor cells to establish a 'foothold' within the recipient. Recent evidence in mice, for example, suggests that among donor-recipient pairs who share one haplotype, donor cell survival is inversely proportional to the NK cell activity of the recipient (Sheng-Tanner and Miller 1992). The immune competence of the recipient may play an important role in the transfusion effect (see figure 1).

Figure 1 *Mononuclear cell microchimerism and the spectrum between graft versus host disease and HLA alloimmunization. The development of microchimerism after allogeneic transfusion may depend upon the number of viable donor leucocytes transfused, the immunocompetence of the recipient, and the HLA similarity between donor and recipient*

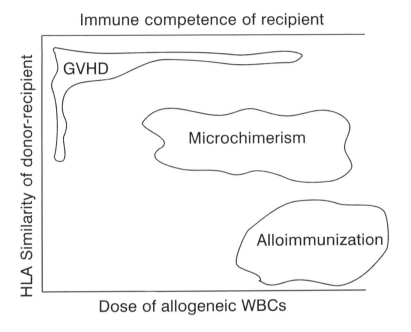

Evidence for microchimerism following selected instances of transplantation and transfusion is irrefutable. The frequent occurrence of postoperative ABO hemolysis in group A recipients of group O solid organ transplants was evidence that transient engraftment of donor B lymphocytes occurred. More recently, studies by Starzl et al. (1992a, 1992b, 1993a) and others (Schlitt et al. 1993) have unequivocally documented donor microchimerism following solid organ transplantation. By using both the polymerase chain reaction to amplify donor genes and immunoperoxidase technology to stain for donor antigens, donor cells have been found in samples of recipient blood, lymph nodes, spleen, skin, heart and other tissue. Remarkably, microchimerism has been demonstrated as long as 29 years after the original transplant. Microchimeric recipients demonstrate donor-specific tolerance but normal reactivity to third party cells in mixed lymphocyte reactions (Starzl et al. 1993b).

Although several studies have documented microchimerism in animals following transfusion, there is limited investigation into the development of microchimerism following allogeneic blood transfusion in humans. Rodents have developed microchimerism (and tolerance) across complete histocompatibility barriers provided that they were first given immunosuppressive conditioning - a situation analogous to human solid organ transplantation. Unconditioned newborn mice demonstrated prolonged circulation of maternal cells whose survival paralleled tolerance towards maternal skin grafts (Zhang and Miller 1993). Human studies of donor lymphocyte survival following HLA *unrelated* transfusions have shown little evidence for microchimerism (Hutchinson et al. 1976, Schechter et al. 1977, Adams et al. 1992). However, different results were found in early studies of blood exchange between mothers and their children. Even with the use of a relatively insensitive assay such as cell karyotyping, prolonged survival of donor cells have been observed. For example, maternal cells transfused to fetuses have been found to circulate in the newborn for up to 4 years (Hutchinson et al. 1971). In addition, fetal cells were shown to persist in the maternal circulation for months after delivery (Whang-Peng et al. 1973).

The development of microchimerism may extend the limits of tolerance or anergy by either central or peripheral mechanisms

There are numerous possible mechanisms by which transient donor mononuclear microchimerism might induce tolerance or anergy to donor antigens (Sykes and Sachs 1988, De Waal and Van Twuyver 1991). For simplicity these can be grouped into two major categories: central tolerance and peripheral anergy. Central tolerance is the development of immunologic tolerance (nonrecognition) as a result of thymic processing. Normal individuals develop tolerance to self antigens as a result of thymic 'education' of immune cells during which self-reactive clones are deleted (Ramsdell and Fowlkes 1990). Transfused donor cells which come to reside in the recipient thymus (or donor cells whose MHC antigens are presented as though they were self in the recipient thymus) may be interpreted by the recipient as self molecules within the thymic environment. Experiments in animals demonstrate that when allogeneic tissue is implanted into the recipient thymus, the recipient becomes tolerant to the donor tissue. For example, prolonged survival of rat orthotopic liver allografts (Campos et al. 1993) or pancreatic allografts (James et al. 1993) has been induced after intrathymic inoculation of donor strain cells into the recipient.

Peripheral anergy refers to a modification of immune responsiveness not dependent upon thymic processing. At least two mechanisms of peripheral anergy have been investigated. One mechanism, referred to as the veto concept, depends upon the immunomodulatory effect of cells derived from transplanted or transfused donor stem cells which become chimeric in the recipient. These donor-origin veto cells can inactivate recipient cytotoxic T cells bearing receptors for antigens present on the veto cell surface (Thomas et al. 1991). Experimental evidence for the existence of veto cells has been found in both rodents and primates following infusion of donor bone marrow (Campos et al. 1993). A number of pretransplant conditioning protocols in animals (Pierce and Watts 1993, Thomas et al. 1989) or in humans (Monaco et al. 1988) have used donor bone marrow as a more effective way to induce microchimerism and peripheral anergy.

A second mechanism of peripheral anergy has explored the phenomenon that allorecognition depends upon presentation of the combination of both alloantigen and specific costimulatory molecules. In the absence of a dual signal, anergy is induced. A growing list of costimulatory molecules including CD80, ICAM-1, LAM-1 are thought to influence antigen recognition. Among sufficiently matched donor-recipient pairs, an adequate dual signal may not be present to induce alloimmunity thus permitting temporary survival of donor cells and the development of anergy towards donor antigens. The recent application of recombinant DNA technology has begun to provide exciting new information on the induction of peripheral tolerance. Several research groups have begun to use recipient cells as a vehicle to introduce selectively allogeneic donor Class I MHC antigens (Wood 1993, Madsen et al. 1988). Recipient marrow cells are transfected with donor Class I MHC genes and reinfused into the recipient. The recipient becomes chimeric with these new cells which induce anergy towards the transfected Class I alloantigens. This experimental model is not too dissimilar from blood transfusion circumstances in which donor cells are disparate at Class I but match at Class II antigens. Experiments such as these hold great promise to define more precisely the events controlling the induction of peripheral anergy.

Future studies

It is very possible that more than one mechanism may account for the observation that in some instances allogeneic transfusions appear to exert an immunosuppressive effect. The development of transient mononuclear cell microchimerism is consistent with the importance of both recipient exposure to viable allogeneic donor leucocytes and HLA similarity between donor and recipient. Our laboratory is currently studying the duration of survival of allogeneic donor mononuclear leucocytes after transfusion among defined HLA donor-recipient pairs. If the donor-recipient HLA conditions can be established which allow for transient donor microchimerism following transfusion, we intend to explore whether or not the development of transient mononuclear cell microchimerism following transfusion will correlate with the development of donor-specific tolerance/anergy. It may be important that future clinical studies seeking to identify the immunomodulatory effects of allogeneic transfusion consider not only the number of viable donor mononuclear cells infused into the recipient, but also consider the HLA relationship between the donor and recipient.

References

Adams P.T., Davenport R.D., Reardon D.A., Roth M.S. (1992) Detection of circulating donor white blood cells in patients receiving multiple blood transfusions, *Blood* 80: 551-555.

Bean M.A., Mickelson E., Yanagida J., Ishioka S., Brannen G.E., Hansen J.A. (1990) Suppressed antidonor MLC responses in renal transplant candidates conditioned with donor-specific transfusions that carry the recipient's noninherited maternal HLA haplotype, *Transplantation* 49: 382-386.

Blajchman M.A., Bardossy L., Carmen R. et al. (1993) Allogeneic blood transfusion-induced enhancement of tumor growth: two animal models showing amelioration by leukodepletion and passive transfer using spleen cells, *Blood* 81: 1880-1882.

Blumberg N., Heal J.M. (1994) Transfusion-associated immunomodulation, in: Anderson K.C., Ness P.M. (eds.) *Scientific Basis of Transfusion Medicine: Implications for Clinical Practice*, W.B. Saunders Co, Philadelphia, pp. 580-597.

Brunson M.E., Alexander J.W. (1990) Mechanisms of transfusion-induced immunosuppression, *Transfusion* 30: 651-658.

Campos L., Alfrey E.J., Posselt A.M. et al. (1993) Prolonged survival of rat orthotopic liver allografts after intrathymic inoculation of donor-strain cells, *Transplantation* 55: 866-870.

Claas F.H.J., Gijbels Y., Van der Velden-de Munck J., Van Rood J.J. (1988) Induction of B cell unresponsiveness to noninherited maternal HLA antigens during fetal life, *Science* 241: 1815-1817.

De Waal L.P., Van Twuyver E. (1991) Blood transfusion and allograft survival: is mixed chimerism the solution for tolerance induction in clinical transplantation?, *Crit Rev Immunol.* 10: 417-425.

Hutchinson D.L., Turner J.H., Schlesinger E.R. (1971) Persistence of donor cells in neonates after fetal and exchange transfusion, *Amer. J. Obstet. Gyn.* 109: 281-284.

Hutchinson I.V. (1986) Suppressor T cells in allogeneic models, *Transplantation* 41: 547-555.

Hutchinson R.M., Sejeny S.A., Fraser I.D., Tovey G.H. (1976) Lymphocyte response to blood transfusion in man: a comparison of different preparations of blood, *Brit. J. Haeme* 33: 105-111.

James T., Ming-Xing J., Chowdhury N.C., Oluwole S.F. (1993) Tolerance induction to rat islet allografts by intrathymic inoculation of donor spleen cells, *Transplantation* 56: 1148-1152.

Jensen L.S., Andersen A.J., Christiansen P.M. et al. (1992) Postoperative infection and natural killer cell function following blood transfusion in patients undergoing elective colorectal surgery, *Brit. J. Surg.* 79: 513-516.

Lagaaij E.L., Hennemann P.H., Ruigrok M. et al. (1989) Effect of one-HLA-DR antigen matched and completely HLA-DR-mismatched blood transfusions on survival of heart and kidney allografts, *N. Engl. J. Med.* 321: 701-705.

Lazda V.T., Rollak R., Mozes M.F., Barber P.L., Jonasson O. (1990) Evidence that HLA Class II disparity is required for the induction of renal allograft enhancement by donor-specific blood transfusions in man, *Transplantation* 49: 1084-1087.

Leivestad T., Thorsby E. (1984) Effects of HLA-haploidentical blood transfusions on donor-specific immune responsiveness, *Transplantation* 37: 175-181.

Madsen J.C., Superina R.A., Wood K.J., Morris P.J. (1988) Immunological unresponsiveness induced by recipient cells transfected with donor MHC genes, *Nature* 332: 161-164.

Meryman H.T. (1989) Transfusion-induced alloimmunization and immunosuppression and the effects of leukocyte depletion, *Transf. Med. Rev.* 3: 180-193.

Monaco A.P., Wood M.L., Maki T. et al. (1988) The use of donor-specific antigen for the induction of immunologic unresponsiveness to experimental and clinical allografts, *Transp. Proc.* 20: 122-130.

Okazaki H., Takahashi M., Miura K. et al. (1985) Effect of buffy coat transfusions in living related and cadaveric renal transplantation, *Transpl. Proc.* 17: 1034-1036.

Pierce G.E., Watts L.M. (1993) Do donor cells function as veto cells in the induction and maintenance of tolerance across an MHC disparity in mixed lymphoid radiation chimeras?, *Transplantation* 55: 882-887.

Quigley R.L., Wood K.J., Morris P.J. (1989) The relative roles of major and minor histocompatibility antigens in the induction of immunologic unresponsiveness by blood transfusion, *Transfusion* 29: 789-793.

Ramsdell F., Fowlkes B.J. (1990) Clonal deletion versus clonal anergy: the role of the thymus in inducing self tolerance, *Science* 248: 1342-1348.

Reed E., Hardy M., Benvenisty A. et al. (1987) Effect of antiidotypic antibodies to HLA on graft survival in renal allograft recipients, *N. Engl. J. Med.* 316: 1450-1455.

Ross W.B., Leaver H.A., Yap P.L., Raab G.M., Su B.H., Carter D.C. (1990) Prostaglandin E2 production by rat peritoneal macrophages: role of cellular and humoral factors in vivo in transfusion-associated immunosuppression, *FEMS Microbiol. Immunol.* 2: 321-325.

Schechter G.P., Whang-Peng J., McFarland W. (1977) Circulation of donor lymphocytes after blood transfusion in man, *Blood* 49: 651-656.

Schlitt J.H., Kanehiro H., Raddatz G. et al. (1993) Persistence of donor lymphocytes in liver allograft recipients, *Transplantation* 56: 1001-1007.

Shelby J., Marushack M.M., Nelson E.W. (1987) Prostaglandin production and suppressor cell induction in transfusion-induced suppression, *Transplantation* 43: 113-116.

Sheng-Tanner X., Miller R.G. (1992) Correlation between lymphocyte-induced donor-specific tolerance and donor cell recirculation, *J. Exp. Med.* 176: 407-413.

Starzl T.E., Demetris A.J., Murase N. et al. (1992a) Cell migration, chimerism, and graft acceptance, *Lancet* 339: 1579-1582.

Starzl T.E., Demetris A.J., Trucco M. et al. (1992b) Systemic chimerism in human female recipients of male livers, *Lancet* 340: 876-877.

Starzl T.E., Demetris A.J., Trucco M. et al. (1993a) Chimerism after liver transplantation for type IV glycogen storage disease and type 1 Gaucher's disease, *N. Engl. J. Med.* 328: 745-749.

Starzl T.E., Demetris A.J., Trucco M. et al. (1993b) Chimerism and donor-specific nonreactivity 27 to 29 years after kidney allotransplantation, *Transplantation* 55: 1272-1277.

Susal C., Terness P., Opelz G. (1990) An experimental model for preventing alloimmunization against platelet transfusions by pretreatment with antibody-coated cells, *Vox Sang.* 59: 209-215.

Sykes M., Sachs D.H. (1988) Mixed allogeneic chimerism as an approach to transplantation tolerance, *Immunol. Today* 9: 23-27.

Terasaki P.I. (1984) The beneficial transfusion effect on kidney graft survival attributed to clonal deletion, *Transplantation* 37: 119-125.

Thomas J.M., Carver M., Cunningham P. et al. (1989) Promotion of incompatible allograft acceptance in rhesus monkeys given posttransplant antithymocyte globulin and donor marrow, *Transplantation* 47: 209-215.

Thomas J.M., Verbanac K.M., Thomas F.T. (1991) The veto mechanism in transplant tolerance, *Transplantation Reviews* 5: 209-229.

Triulzi D.J., Heal J.M., Blumberg N. (1990) Transfusion-induced immunomodulation and its clinical consequences, in: Nance S.J. (ed.) *Transfusion Medicine in the 1990's*, American Association of Blood Banks, Arlington, VA, pp. 1-33.

Van Aken, W.G. (1989) Does perioperative blood transfusion promote tumor growth?, *Transf. Med. Rev.* 3: 243-252.

Van Rood J.J., Claas F.H.J. (1990) The influence of allogeneic cells on the human T and B cell repertoire, *Science* 248: 1388-1393.

Van Twuyer E., Mooijaart R.J.D., Ten Berge I.J.M. et al. (1991) Pretransplant blood transfusions revisited, *N. Engl. J. Med*. 325: 1210-1213.

Whang-Peng J., Leikin S., Harris C., Lee E., Sites J. (1973) Transplacental passage of fetal leukocytes into the maternal blood, *Proc. Soc. Exp. Biol. Med*. 142: 50-53.

Wood K.J. (1993) The induction of tolerance to alloantigens using MHC class I molecules, *Curr. Opinion Immunol*. 5: 759-762.

Zhang L., Miller R.G. (1993) The correlation of prolonged survival of maternal skin grafts with the presence of naturally transferred maternal T cells, *Transplantation* 56: 918-921.

Technical Aspects of Leucocyte Depletion

7 | T. Nishimura, S. Oka and N. Yamawaki

Introduction

Table 1 summarizes a history of filters for blood transfusion.

Table 1 *History of filters for blood transfusion*

Generation	Removal target	Filter materials
1st	Micro-aggregates	Screen filter (pore size: 170-240 μm)
2nd	Micro-aggregates	Screen filter (pore size: ca 40 μm) and/or Depth filter
3rd	Leucocytes	Mass of fine fibres (fibre diameter: 10-20 μm)
4th	Leucocytes	Non-woven web of ultrafine fibres (fibre diameter: 1-2 μm)

With generation advancement, it has been necessary to remove smaller impurities with higher efficiency. In order to meet this advancement, filter materials have evolved from surface filters with large pore sizes to depth filters having small pores.

Table 2 summarizes size, specific gravity and concentration of blood cells. Figure 1 shows the order of blood cell adhesiveness against materials (Rabinowitz 1964).

Table 2 *Size, specific gravity and concentration of blood cells*

Blood cells	Size (μm)	Specific gravity	Concentration (/μL)
Red cells	6-9	1,093-1,096	$4\text{-}6\times10^6$
Leucocyte	6-20	1,055-1,092	$3\text{-}8\times10^3$
Granulocyte	10-15	1,087-1,092	(4×10^3)
Monocyte	13-20	1,065-1,068	(4×10^2)
Lymphocyte	6-12	1,055-1,070	(2×10^3)
Platelet	2-4	1,040-1,058	$1\text{-}4\times10^5$

Figure 1 *Adhesiveness of blood cells against materials*

Red Cell ≤ Lymphocyte ‹ ‹ Platelet ‹ Granulocyte ≤ Monocyte

Considering this information, it seems to be difficult to remove contaminated lymphocytes from red cell products, because the difference in size and adhesiveness between lymphocytes and red cells is small. It seems to be impossible to remove contaminated lymphocytes from platelet products, because platelets are far more adhesive against materials than lymphocytes.

In this paper, we demonstrate how 4th generation filters have solved these difficult problems and express our opinion for the direction of future filter development.

Blood cell entrapment characteristics of 4th generation filters

Materials for 4th generation filters are non-woven webs comprising ultrafine fibres of 1-2 μm diameter (Watanabe and Rikumaru 1984, Nishimura et al. 1989). As shown in Figure 2, the leucocyte removal ability of fibre filters are enhanced with thinner fibre diameters and this shows a steep elevation around 3μm diameter.

Figure 2 *Average fibre diameter and leucocyte removal ability of non-woven web filters*

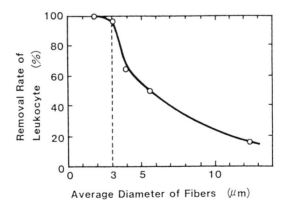

Figures 3 and 4 show electron micrographs of leucocytes trapped by 4th and 3rd generation filters.

Figure 3 *Electron micrographs of leucocytes trapped by 4th generation filter* A, *and 3rd generation filters* B *and* C

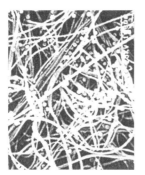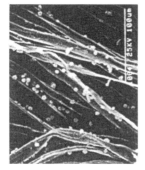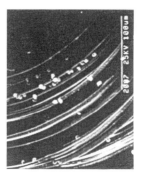

Figure 4 *Electron micrographs (large magnification) of leucocytes trapped by 4th generation filter* A

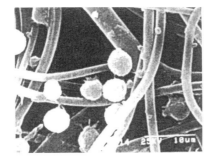

In the case of 3rd generation filters, each leucocyte is in contact with a fibre at one point, while in the case of 4th generation filters, each leucocyte is in contact with fibres through multi-points near a fibre cross-over point. It is thus supposed that the adsorption power of leucocytes to fibres in 4th generation filters is stronger than that in 3rd generation filters.

In addition, the number of leucocyte adsorption points in 3rd generation filters are estimated to be proportional to the surface area of fibres which relates to square of reciprocal of fibre-diameter, while that in 4th generation filters (the number of fibre cross-over points) is estimated to be proportional to the cube of a reciprocal of fibre-diameter. Furthermore, fibre cross-over points are formed more efficiently in non-woven webs than in a cotton-like mass of fibres.

Comparative features between 4th and 3rd generation filters are summarized in Table 3.

Table 3 *Comparison between 4th and 3rd generation filter*

	4th	3rd
Number of attachment point per trapped leucocyte	2-3	1
Fibre diameter dependency of adsorption point number per unit fibre weight	$\left[\dfrac{1}{fibre\ diameter}\right]^{3+\alpha}$	$\left[\dfrac{1}{fibre\ diameter}\right]^{2}$

It is indicated that the 4th generation filter has an overwhelming number of adsorption points for leucocyte per unit fibre weight with reinforced adsorption power at the point as compared with the 3rd generation filter.

Figure 5 *Logarithmic residual rate of granulocyte, lymphocyte and platelet (PLT) after filtration against the thickness (X:mm) of the non-woven webs*

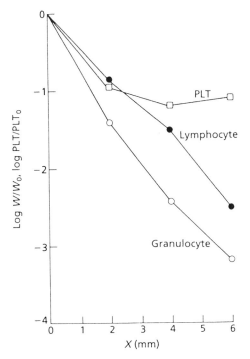

Figure 5 shows the residual rate of granulocytes, lymphocytes and platelets after filtration of red cell concentrate preserved for 3 days at 4°C, plotted against the thickness of the non-woven webs (Oka et al. 1993). The residual rate of both granulocytes and lymphocytes decreased logarithmically against the thickness of the non-woven webs with larger slope for the former. This suggests that both granulocytes and lymphocytes are of relatively uniform mass concerning adsorption and that granulocytes are more adsorptive than lymphocytes. On the contrary, about 10% of platelets passed through the filter irrespective of its thickness. The residual platelets seemed to have lost their adhesiveness to the material during preservation for 3 days at 4°C. By performing the analytical procedures as shown in Figure 5, removal mechanisms of blood cells by filtration have become elucidated under various blood conditions with various materials.

Most of leucocyte removal behaviours of 4th generation filters can be explained by a concept that leucocytes are entrapped through an adsorption mechanism. For example, the decreased leucocyte removal performance with increased amount of filtered blood is explained by decreased number of free adsorption points caused by covering with adsorbed leucocytes. The slightly decreased leucocyte removal performance in response to elevated Ht-value in red cell concentrate is attributed to inhibited leucocyte approach to the adsorption point due to the elevated red cell concentration. The slightly reduced leucocyte removal performance in response to accelerated blood flow is attributable to partial detachment of adsorbed leucocytes due to accelerated share stress.

In the case of quite fresh blood, the transformation capacity of granulocytes may have great influence on their entrapment in the filters. Some papers reported results of experiment using metabolic inhibitors (Oka et al. 1993, Sasakawa et al. 1989, Dzik 1993). Possible interaction between granulocytes and platelets have also been reported (Dzik 1993, Steneker and Biewenga 1991). Further studies are needed for more detailed analyses.

Control of blood cell adsorption by surface modification

Entrapment of blood cells by 4th generation filters are mainly obtained by an adsorption mechanism. Adsorption of blood cells on materials largely depend on the chemical composition of material surfaces. Figure 6 shows effects of HE-X polymer coating on blood cell pass ratios. HE-X is a copolymer of hydrophilic monomer and positively charged monomer (X: Content of charged monomer in %). The HE-5 coated filter allows better platelet permeation while efficiently entrapping leucocytes. On the basis of this technology, we have developed leucocyte removal filters for platelet products (Sekiguchi and Takahashi 1989). In addition, HE-20 coated filters having larger amounts of positive charge are able to entrap both leucocytes and platelets with high efficiency. On the basis of this technology we are developing high performance filters for red cell products.

In the field of biomedical material science, material design research for the separation of blood components is making rapid progress (Nishimura 1993). For example, precise separation of B and T lymphocytes has been achieved by a material having a microphage separated structure similar to an aggregated state of membrane proteins in cell membranes (Kataoka 1993). In plasma purification treatments by extracorporeal circulation, selective and specific removals of malignant substances using synthetic and biological ligands have been developed for practical use (Nishimura 1993). It is also expected that these technologies will be applied to the field of transfusion and bring about dramatic progress.

Figure 6 *Effects of HE-X coating on pass ratios of leucocyte and platelet*

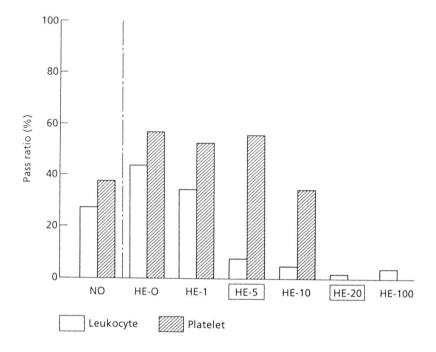

Figure 7 *Closed system for whole blood filtration*

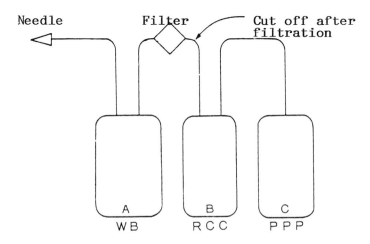

System design

In the practical use of leucocyte removal filters, the entire system including connection tubing and blood bags also play an important role. Recently, advantages of pre-storage leucocyte removal have been widely recognized, and various types of closed systems have been developed.

Figure 7 illustrates a closed system for whole blood treatment designed by Asahi Medical (Takahashi et al. 1992). This system has the advantage of not requiring centrifugation of the filter, and ensures leucocyte removal from all products.

Conclusion

The design of specific physical structure using non-woven web of ultrafine fibres has contributed much to the breakthrough from 3rd generation filters to the 4th. The development of the 5th generation filters will most probably depend on highly advanced design of chemical structure of filter surfaces. System developments including closed system will be further elaborated. By encouraging interdisciplinary researches between medical science and engineering, it is expected that this field will make aggressive progress.

References

Dzik S. (1993) Leukodepletion blood filters: filter design and mechanisms of leukocyte removal, *Transfusion Medicine Reviews* 7: 65-77.

Kataoka K. (1993) Development of polymeric adsorbents for separation of lymphocyte subpopulations, in: Sekiguchi S. (ed.) *Clinical Application of Leukocyte Depletion*, Blackwell Scientific Publications, Oxford, pp. 130-137.

Miyamoto M. et al. (1989) Leukocyte-poor platelet concentrates at the bedside by filtration though Sepacell-PL, *Vox Sang.* 57: 164-167.

Nishimura T. et al. (1989) Advanced methods for leucocyte removal by blood filtration, in: Borozvic B. (ed.) *The Role of Leucocyte Depletion in Blood Transfusion Practice*, Blackwell Scientific Publications, Oxford, pp. 35-40

Nishimura T. (1993) Polymer materials for blood purification, in: Tsuruta T. et al. (eds.) *Biomedical Applications of Polymeric Materials*, CRC Press, Boca Raton, pp. 191-218.

Oka S. et al. (1993) Mechanism of leukocyte removal with fibers, in: Sekiguchi S. (ed.) *Clinical Application of Leukocyte Depletion*, Blackwell Scientific Publications, Oxford, pp. 105-118.

Rabinowitz Y. (1964) Separation of lymphocytes, polymorphonuclear leukocytes and monocytes on glass columns, including tissue culture observations, *Blood* 23: 811.

Sasakawa S. et al (1989) The use of Sepacell PL for platelet concentrates, in: Brozovic B. (ed.) *The Role of Leucocyte Depletion in Blood Transfusion Practice*, Blackwell Scientific Publications, Oxford, pp. 56-63.

Sekiguchi S. and Takahashi T.A. (1989) Leucocyte-depleted blood products and their clinical usefulness, in: Borozvic B. (ed.) *The Role of Leucocyte Depletion in Blood Transfusion Practice*, Blackwell Scientific Publications, Oxford, pp. 26-34.

Steneker I. and Biewenga J. (1991) Histologic and immunohisto-chemical studies on the preparation of white cell-poor red cell concentrates: The filtration process using three different polyester filters, *Transfusion.* 31: 40-46.

Takahashi T.A. et al. (1992) Evaluation of a new leukocyte removal filter, the R-S350, in a closed system, *Jpn. J. Transfus. Med.* 38: 401-407.

Watanabe H. and Rikumaru H. (1984) *U.S. Patent* 4,701,267.

Clinical Experience of White Cell Reduction in Blood Components: An Overview

8 | G. Sirchia

Introduction

The transfusion of leucocyte-reduced (LR) red blood cells (RBC) and platelet concentrates (PC) is widely used, particularly in some specialties such as haematology and oncology. This practice was originally promoted by the ability of LR-RBC in preventing the occurrence of non hemolytic, febrile transfusion reactions (NHFTR) in patients alloimmunized to the human leucocyte antigen (HLA) system (Brittingham and Chaplin 1957). Further investigation has shown that the use of LR blood components involves a number of additional benefits to the recipients, such as decrease of the frequency of alloimmunization to HLA (Sirchia et al. 1986, Andreu et al. 1988, Oksanen et al. 1991) and prevention of transmission of cytomegalovirus (CMV) (Lamberson and Dock 1992), while other possible advantages are still under evaluation, including the reduction of transfusion-induced immunomodulation that has been associated with increased occurrence of infection and tumor recurrence in transfused surgical patients (Nowak and Ponsky 1984, Nathanson et al. 1985, Blumberg and Heal 1987, Voogt et al. 1987, Blumberg et al. 1990, Triulzi et al. 1992).

A more general use of LR blood components has been favored by technical improvements of filters for white cell reduction, which are currently capable of decreasing the number of white cells present in RBC from average values around $3,000 \times 10^6$ to less than 3×10^6 per unit (3-4 log reduction) (Masse et al. 1992, Pietersz et al. 1992, Rebulla et al. 1993). Although filters for leucoreduction of PC are slightly less effective, LR-PC containing less than 5×10^6 white cells per platelet transfusion can be easily prepared with current filters from different manufacturers (Sintnicolaas and Van Putten 1993). While the level of 5×10^8 white cells per unit is the maximum value recommended for the prevention of NHFTR (Widmann 1993), the smaller value of 5×10^6 white cells per unit has been given as a threshold value that should not be exceeded to prevent transmission of CMV and alloimmunization to HLA (Fisher et al. 1985, Widmann 1993). Some uncertainty on the latter level derives from the absence of definitive scientific evidence on the smallest number of white cells capable of causing complications to the recipient and of accurate methods for counting very low numbers of white cells.

In spite of the significant achievements that have been possible by leucoreduction of blood components through filtration, several issues have not been fully clarified yet.

In this overview the following aspects will be considered: (1) clinical indications; (2) level of leucoreduction required; (3) quality control; (4) filtration in the laboratory *versus* filtration at the patient's bedside; (5) pre-storage *versus* post-storage white cell reduction. Finally, (6) perspectives for the near future will be discussed.

Clinical indications to the use of LR blood components

Prevention of NHFTR

The best defined and most commonly accepted indication to the use of LR blood components is the prevention of NHFTR, a complication mainly caused by anti-HLA antibodies (Décary et al. 1984, Brubaker 1990). Basic data supporting this indication have been reported by Brittingham and Chaplin (1957), who published a study showing that NHFTR is due to alloimmunization to donor white cells and platelets. In a subsequent study, Perkins et al. (1966) found a relation between the number of white cells transfused and the temperature rise associated with NHFTR.

Our clinical experience with leucoreduction began in the 70's, when we started a transfusion program for a large group of homozygous ß-thalassaemics. These patients require chronic blood transfusion throughout their lifetime, that currently can last more than 20-30 years (Zurlo et al. 1989). Most patients receive 2 units of RBC every 2-4 weeks (Cao et al. 1992), and approximately 2/3 of them develop anti-HLA antibodies if transfused with non-LR RBC. In 1980 the majority of our patients were given buffy-coat free RBC, which resulted in approximately 60% of them developing NHFTR in 11% of transfusions. In subsequent years, different filters and filtration techniques were used that progressively allowed the achievement of lower and lower levels of white cell count in leucoreduced RBC. This was paralleled by a decrease of NHFTR that now occur in 2-3% of our thalassaemic patients and in less than 1% of transfusions (Sirchia et al. 1990).

A similarly impressive reduction of NHFTR has not been obtained in recipients of LR-PC (Mangano et al. 1991, Mintz 1991, Goodnough et al. 1993). This has been reported in recent studies performed both in the general population of PC recipients and in groups of patients with previous NHFTR (reactors). Table 1 reports a summary of some comparative studies together with previous data obtained by Décary and coworkers in recipients of standard PC pools, presented as historical reference data (Décary et al. 1984). Table 1 shows that leucoreduction by filtration, although capable of slightly reducing the incidence of NHFTR in some studies, was inferior to single donor (apheresis) PC in one study (Chambers et al. 1990), and was associated with a paradoxically increased occurrence in others (Goodnough et al. 1993, Riccardi et al. 1993). It should be pointed out that in most studies patients given unfiltered PC were different from those treated with filtered PC, which can create some difficulty in the interpretation of these data. However, these studies clearly indicate that the efficacy of filtration leucoreduction of stored PC in decreasing the frequency of NHFTR in PC recipients is not as impressive as it is in recipients of RBC.

Table 1 *Frequency of reactions reported after the transfusion of different types of filtered and non-filtered PC to general patient populations (A) and to patients with previous reactions when transfused with standard PC (reactors) (B)*

Author	Year	Type of PC	Number of transfusions	Number of reactions	Transfusion reaction rate (%)
(A) General population					
Décary	1984	Standard PC	795	22	2.8
Goodnough	1993	Standard PC	1901	32	1.7
		Filtered PC	1704	90	5.3
Riccardi	1993	Buffy-coat PC	1476	7	0.47
		Filtered buffy-coat PC	2014	24	1.19
(B) Reactors					
Chambers	1990	Standard PC	583	125	21.4
		Single donor PC	438	37	8.4
Mangano	1991	Standard PC	202	55	27.2
		Filtered PC	206	40	19.4
Goodnough	1993	Standard PC	152	20	13
		Filtered PC	152	15	10

A clue to the interpretration of the cause for this finding comes from recent studies showing that cytokines are released by white cells into the platelet suspending medium during PC storage (Mintz 1991, Muylle et al. 1993, Stack and Snyder 1994) and that early white cell removal can prevent cytokine release (Muylle and Peetermans 1994). It is known that certain cytokines including interleukin-1ß, interleukin-6, interleukin-8 and tumor necrosis factor can mediate the onset of symptoms frequently reported during NHFTR (Dzik 1992, Muylle and Peetermans 1994). The observation that the release of these cytokines in PC is particularly evident from the third to the fifth day of storage (Stack and Snyder 1994) is in accordance with our findings that most reactions occur towards the end of the platelet storage period (Riccardi et al. 1994, unpublished).

Definitive conclusions on the role of PC leucoreduction in the prevention of NHFTR following platelet transfusion cannot be drawn at the moment. The current level of information supports the need for further study in this area. For the time being, we believe that, if filtration is used with the goal of preventing NHFTR, platelet filters should be used only with PC stored for less than three days, and the filtered PC should be administered only to patients with anti-HLA antibodies in the serum, showing repeated NHFTR occurring also with fresh platelets.

Prevention of virus transmission

It is reasonable to expect that leucoreduction of blood units could prevent the transmission of viral infections caused by leucocyte-restricted viruses. This has been definitely proven for CMV (Verdonk et al. 1985, Gilbert et al. 1989, De

Graan et al. 1989, Bowden et al. 1991, Eisenfeld et al. 1992). The recent 'Guide to the preparation, use and quality assurance of blood components' published in 1992 by the Council of Europe indicates that the use of LR blood components is an acceptable alternative to components prepared from units given by anti-CMV negative subjects (Council of Europe 1992). Similarly, a new indication to the use of LR-RBC as a means of preventing CMV transmission has been proposed for inclusion in the forthcoming 16th Edition of the Standards for Blood Banks and Transfusion Services of the American Association of Blood Banks (AABB) (Standards Committee 1993). The practical advantages of using leucoreduction instead of anti-CMV screening of blood donors are particularly evident in large urban areas where the prevalence of CMV seropositivity in the donor population can be very high (Tegtmeier 1989). However, the relative cost-effectiveness of these two strategies needs to be determined.

In addition to the above data on CMV, some evidence has been gathered indicating that leucoreduction could prevent also the transmission of human T-cell lymphotropic virus (HTLV), an agent associated with the development of adult T-cell leukaemia and tropical spastic paraparesis (Okochi and Sato 1986, Al et al. 1993). This agent does not seem to be particularly diffused outside certain geographic areas including Japan. However, concern caused by the possibility of transfusion-induced transmission prompted the implementation of mandatory screening of blood donors for anti-HTLV antibodies in several Western countries, in addition to Japan.

As far as HIV is concerned, this virus circulates not only into intact leucocytes, but also in leucocyte fragments and free in plasma. It is therefore unlikely that leucoreduction, which cannot remove leucocyte fragments (Engelfriet et al. 1975, Ramos et al. 1994), although capable of significantly decreasing the viral load (Bruisten et al. 1990), could be sufficient to prevent the transmission of the virus (Rawal et al. 1989).

Prevention of HLA alloimmunization

Although HLA antigens are present both on platelets and leucocytes, it has been reported that pure platelets cannot induce primary alloimmunization to HLA (Claas et al. 1981). Additional studies have elucidated the key role of antigen presenting cells (APC) of donor origin (as opposed to recipient's APC) in inducing the production of anti-HLA antibodies. Therefore, protocols developed to prevent anti-HLA alloimmunization are based on the reduction of donor APC.

During the last two decades, newly diagnosed, previously untransfused homozygous ß-thalassaemia patients admitted to the Department of Pediatrics of our Hospital have been transfused with RBC depleted of leucocytes with the best available technique, with the aim of showing if this could prevent the development of anti-HLA antibodies. The study protocol required the transfusion of fresh (1-5 days old) RBC in which no white cells could be counted with the most sensitive counting techniques that have progressively become available throughout the study period. Before the recent development of methods based on the Nageotte counting chamber, which permit a reasonably accurate detection of 1 white cell per microliter, (or 300,000 white cells in a 300 mL RBC unit) (Rebulla and Dzik 1994), residual white cells in filtered RBC used in this study were counted with a modification of the traditional manual method based on the Bürker's chamber (Sirchia et al. 1986). The theoretical lower limit of detection of this method is higher than that using the Nageotte chamber. In fact, the lowest possible detection of 1 white cell in two sides (1.8 μL) of a Bürker's chamber after 1:10 sample dilution corresponds to 5.5 white cells per microliter of native sample, or 1.65×10^6 white cells in a 300 mL RBC unit. Our protocol required that all RBC units used in the study were examined for their white cell count and that filtered RBC could be used for the study only if no white cells could be detected by the counting method. Therefore, also in consideration of the inaccuracy related to the detection of very few events in counting methods (Dumont 1991), we can reasonably assume that all our patients received less than 5×10^6 white cells per transfusion, which on average consisted of 1 and 2 RBC units before and after the age of 4 respectively. So far, 22 of the 27 patients enrolled received each more than 80 RBC transfusions. Recently reviewed results of this study indicate that 2 of 14 patients enrolled in the leuco-'free' arm developed anti-HLA antibodies after 50 transfusions, compared to 9 of 13 thalassaemics transfused with buffy-coat depleted RBC (controls). This study shows that primary HLA alloimmunization can be significantly delayed and possibly prevented in a great proportion of pediatric recipients of RBC units containing less than 5×10^6 white cells per transfusion. However, it also shows that even such small numbers of white cells are capable in the long run to trigger a primary immune response to HLA in some patients, thus suggesting that extremely efficient filters need to be employed for preventing alloimmunization to HLA.

The theoretical implications of our results are much more important than the practical ones, since NHFTR in chronic recipients of RBC can be easily prevented with the use of several filters present in the market, regardless of patient alloimmunization to HLA. In contrast, this is not the case if the negative effects of anti-HLA alloimmunization are considered in oncohaematological recipients of standard RBC and PC. In fact, approximately 30-40% of these subjects develop anti-HLA antibodies, which can decrease the effectiveness of platelet transfusion, and one half of them eventually become refractory to random-donor platelet support (Schiffer 1991). Although methods to provide effective platelets to these patients are available, based on donor HLA selection or platelet crossmatching, both approaches are very expensive and require significant organizational efforts. In addition, even the best methods have a failure rate of approximately 25%. This can cause a significant risk of serious bleeding, that can be fatal in some cases. Therefore, prevention of anti-HLA alloimmunization in haematological recipients of RBC and PC, in addition to the theoretical interest related to its biological relevance, has important practical implications for a large group of transfusion recipients. Leucoreduction through filtration is not the only method currently being investigated to prevent the development of anti-HLA antibodies and, in turn, refractoriness to random-donor platelet support. The use of single-donor platelets and of UV-irradiation represent possible alternative strategies currently under investigation (Andreu et al. 1992). A definitive answer on the relative merits of different methods to prevent or reduce the incidence of alloimmunization to HLA is expected to become available after the conclusions of the ongoing Trial to Reduce Alloimmunization to Platelets (TRAP), a large multicenter investigation performed in the United States (Schiffer 1991).

Conflicting opinions have been presented on the need for or appropriateness of leucoreduction for all PC (International Forum 1992, Wenz 1992). This seems to some authors potentially useful particularly in leukaemics and in other chronically transfused patients suffering from haematological disorders who show a significant risk of developing refractoriness to random donor platelets. However, at the time of this writing (March 1994) neither the 15th edition of the 'Standards for Blood Banks and Transfusion Services' of the AABB (Widmann 1993) nor the 'Guide to the preparation, use and quality assurance of blood components' published by the Council of Europe (1992) contain a mandatory indication to the use of LR-RBC and LR-PC in leukaemics or other oncohaematology recipients to prevent development of alloimmunization to HLA. Rather, a proposal for inclusion into the forthcoming edition of the former document just states that 'when [leucocyte-reduced red blood cells are] *intended for the prevention of* cytomegalovirus infection or *HLA alloimmunization*, the component should be prepared by a method known to reduce the leucocyte number in the final component to less than $5x10^6$' (italics and text in brackets added) (Standards Committee 1993). Similarly, the European document includes just a sentence reading: 'When leucocyte depleted platelets are used, the risk of HLA alloimmunisation is minimal' (Council of Europe 1992). The lack of precise recommendations in certain important pathologies such as leukaemia reflects the limited information available on the most appropriate time and technique for leucoreduction (pre-storage *versus* post-storage) and on the limited number of studies on its cost-effectiveness, as determined in large, prospective, controlled, randomized clinical trials. It is hoped that the TRAP can provide additional information also in regard to these aspects.

Level of leucoreduction required

The continuous improvement of leucoreduction techniques may have generated some confusion regarding the use of the terms leucocyte-depleted, -reduced, -removed, -poor and -free. Occasionally, the same term has been used for defining blood components with greatly different white cell numbers. The 9th edition (1985) of the Technical Manual of the AABB reports that 'the designation "Leucocyte-Poor Red Blood Cells" implies removal of at least 70% of the original white cells and retention of at least 70% of the original red cells' (p. 41) (Widmann 1985). The current, 11th edition (1993) reports the following definition, which includes two levels of leucoreduction: 'the designation "Leucocyte-Reduced Red Blood Cells" applies to those RBCs prepared by a method known to reduce the leucocyte number in the final component to less than $5x10^8$ and to retain at least 80% of the original rbcs. This component is intended to prevent nonhemolytic febrile transfusion reactions. If LR-RBC [leucocyte-reduced RBC] are intended for other purposes, such as preventing CMV infection or [HLA] alloimmunization, the method should reduce the leucocytes in the final component to less than 5×10^6' (p. 59, text in brackets added) (Walker 1993). These definitions depend in part on the developments of new and more effective techniques for leucoreduction, and in part on new information on levels of leucoreduction necessary and sufficient to prevent specific complications. The levels of 5×10^8 and 5×10^6 that are commonly cited in papers, reviews and recommendations define two different technological domains. The former refers to methods not employing filters, based on buffy-coat removal or cell washing (Sirchia et al. 1988), which are generally considered sufficient for the prevention of most NHFTR, with the exception of some heavily immunized recipients, who require more extensive leucoreduction. The latter is consistently achievable with many current commercial filters (Rebulla et al. 1993), and has been clearly associated with the prevention of CMV transmission (Gilbert et al. 1989). Moreover, this level is capable of reducing the frequency of primary HLA alloimmunization not only in patients on chronic RBC substitution (Sirchia et al. 1986) but also in recipients of RBC and PC (Andreu et al. 1988).

The availability of more and more effective filters prompted the expectation that the development of transfusion-associated graft *versus* host disease (TA-GVHD), which can occur and is almost invariably fatal not only in immunocompromised recipients but also in some immunocompetent patients (Thaler et al. 1989, Sanders and Graeber 1990, Anderson et al. 1991, Moroff and Luban 1992) might be prevented by leucoreduction. Although this is tenable in principle, this possibility has been dismissed for the present time and level of technology following some cases reported in the literature on the occurrence of TA-GVHD in recipients of blood components leucoreduced with highly effective filters (Heim et al. 1991, Akahoshi et al. 1992).

Quality control

The assay
Quality control of leucoreduction is a difficult area, mainly because what is being searched for (i.e. the residual leucocytes) is largely missing. The theoretical aspects of counting small numbers of events have been considered in several publications (Dacie and Lewis 1991, Dumont 1991). Some recommendations require that 1% of units, with a minimum of 4 per month are tested (Council of Europe 1992). With the current level of leucoreduction (Pietersz et al. 1992, Rebulla et al. 1993) which can not infrequently leave a total of 3-5 white cells to be counted in an entire Nageotte chamber (Masse et al. 1992), one could argue on the rationale of this approach. However, counting all or a large proportion of units is generally considered not cost-effective, due to the high cost of the counting procedure. The Central Indiana Regional Blood Center, Indianapolis, USA, reported a cost per counting procedure with the Nageotte chamber of US$ 27.36 (Anonymous 1994).

Figure 1 *Observed vs expected leucocyte concentration detected with the 3% PFA method in RBC suspensions containing 0.005-5 leucocytes/μL. The solid line represents the ideal regression*

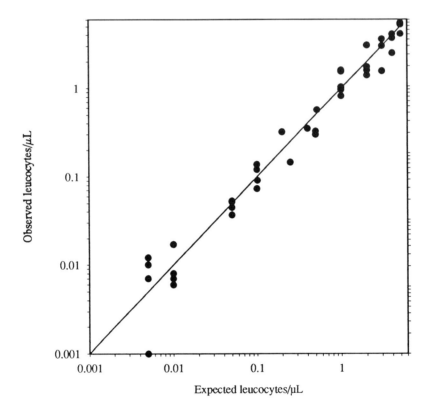

Non-morphological methods based on radiometric techniques (Vos et al. 1987, Wester et al. 1990) or on DNA amplification through the polymerase chain reaction have been developed (Rawal et al. 1989), but their use in routine conditions is impractical. A new method capable of collecting larger numbers of events (leucocytes) that seems to offer a lower limit of detection of 0.05 white cells per microliter has been developed (Prati et al. 1994). This method uses a simple 3% paraformaldehyde (PFA) solution described for the preservation of white cells used in molecular biology techniques (Kiessling et al. 1993). In this procedure 10 mL of filtered RBC are first diluted 1:5 with the 3% PFA solution. The white cells are then pelleted and resuspended in 500 μL of medium. The procedure causes a 20-fold concentration of residual white cells, which are finally counted in a Nageotte chamber. This method has been validated only for 1 day old RBC, and its reliability must be further investigated in large-scale exercises. Nonetheless, the regression reported in Figure 1, which was obtained at very low leucocyte counts, indicates that this method should be sufficiently accurate at leucoreduction levels

approximating 4 log, ie one leucoreduction log more compared to currently validated methods (Masse et al. 1992, Moroff et al. 1994, Rebulla and Dzik 1994). For
the sake of a better comparison of the results that can be obtained with different
methods, Table 2 reports the characteristics of some chambers and methods used
to determine the residual number of leucocytes in LR-RBC. The confidence intervals of the numbers of residual leucocytes that are obtained with different
methods have been reported in the literature (Dumont 1991).

Table 2 *Characteristics of chambers and methods used to determine the residual
number of leucocytes in leucoreduced RBC. A comparison of expected white cell counts
using different counting chambers with different methods at different leucocyte concentrations is also given*

Author (year)	Type of counting chamber	Volume that can be examined in one chamber (μL, 2 grids)	Ratio of native sample to counting fluid	No. of white cells expected to be counted in one chamber (2 grids) with native samples containing:		No. of white cells in a 300 mL unit if 5[*] leuco-cytes per chamber (2 grids) are counted
				1 WBC/μL	5 WBC/μL	
Sirchia (1986)	Bürker	1.8	1:10	0.18	0.9	8.3×10^6
Greenwalt (1990)	not reported	5.4[**]	1:1	5.4	27	277×10^3
Masse (1992)	Nageotte	100	1:10	10	50	150×10^3
Dzik[***] (1993)	Nageotte	100	1:5	20	100	75×10^3
Masse (1992)	Nageotte	100	1:1	100	500	15×10^3
Masse (1992)	Nageotte	100	2:1	200	1000	7.5×10^3
Prati (1994)	Nageotte	100	20:1	2000	10000	0.75×10^3

* Since the error of counting approximates the square root of the number of events counted, 5
events per chamber are presented as an arbitrary example of minimum count that should be obtained in order to prevent too large counting errors.
** In this method three hemocytometers (chambers) are used.
*** Reported in Rebulla and Dzik (1994).

The process
The lower limit of accurate detection and the precision of the method used for
counting residual white cells are key factors in quality control of leucoreduced
blood components. However, discussing these factors does not exhaust the subject of quality control (Anonymous 1992). It is important also to consider additional factors that can influence the level of leucoreduction obtained, such as
those related to the variability in filter production and in the process of filtration.
Strategies must be defined that reduce these effects to a minimum. Controlling
the variability in filter production belongs to good manufacturing practice, which
is routinely performed by renowned manufacturers. The end user of the filters

can control the quality of the filter by checking the level of leucoreduction obtained with a small number of filters (5-10) of each new lot.

In addition to good manufacturing practice at production and control of the filter's performance in each new lot, it is mandatory that a written version of the procedure of filtration is available to the staff in the format of a standard operative procedure, that technologists are properly trained and that the filtration performance of the staff is monitored at regular intervals by determining the white cell residuals (as well as the RBC or platelet yields) obtained by different technologists. While controlling the staff performance in the laboratory is not a difficult task, some arguments have been raised on the possibility of doing so for filtration procedures performed at the patient's bedside.

Filtration in the laboratory *versus* filtration at the bedside

Opponents and advocates of bedside filtration have been confronting their respective arguments in a long lasting debate. The main points under discussion relate to (1) the possibility of performing a reliable quality control procedure at the bedside, and even if this is feasible, to (2) the concern that once the quality control has been completed, the blood component has already been transfused to the recipient, with the risk of 'shutting the stable door after the horse has gone'. In regard to the first point, we offer some data collected in our Institution to support our view that under specific conditions the quality of bedside filtration is not inferior to that performed in the laboratory. To address this important question, we investigated the feasibility and reliability of quality control of bedside filtration in our haematology outpatient clinic. In this setting, the nurses involved in blood transfusion were trained in the use of bedside filters, and their performance was controlled by counting the number of residual white cells in segments of the transfusion set, collected from the tubing severed at 5-25 cm below the drip chamber. A similar experiment was performed also in the laboratory, where the segments were examined in parallel to samples collected from the bag containing the filtered RBC. The results of these studies showed that there was no significant difference in the number of white cells counted in the segments collected at the bedside *versus* those collected in the laboratory, and that both were not significantly different from those obtained in the bag containing the RBC filtered in the laboratory (Sirchia et al. 1994). From these results we concluded that the process of RBC filtration at the patient's bedside can be equal in quality to that performed in the laboratory, at least in clinical settings such as haematology and oncology departments, where blood transfusion is common practice, and if simple training is provided to the nursing staff.

As far as the second argument is concerned, choosing to count residual white cells in all filtered units with validated methods (that, unfortunately, are time consuming), is unfeasible in most settings, independently from the place where leucoreduction is performed. Therefore, also the vast majority of units filtered in the laboratory are transfused to the patient without an evaluation of the number of residual white cells.

In our opinion, the point on quality control should not be viewed in terms of bedside *versus* laboratory filtration, but rather in regard to the indication for which leucoreduction is required. It is in fact evident that exceeding the white cell threshold for CMV transmission in a bone marrow transplant recipient or in a low-weight premature neonate carries a significantly greater risk of morbidity and mortality than passing the number of white cells capable of evoking a NHFTR in a chronic recipient. Thus, in the former indication it seems prudent and wise to count all units (that should be filtered in the laboratory), whereas in the latter bedside filtration and a quality control program similar to the one developed in our Institution do not seem to cause significant risk to the recipients. These considerations apply to the current level of knowledge, and should be adapted to the rapidly evolving technology and information available in this area. A key factor in this regard is the proportion of units that need to be filtered.

For the time being, we believe that bedside filtration is safe and feasible for specific indications, and that it can entail significant advantages in specific settings, such as large thalassaemia centers of the mediterranean area, where not infrequently each of several hundred patients needs to be transfused with 2-3 units of filtered RBC every 2-4 weeks .

It might seem that bedside filtration could favour a loss of control of filtration procedures and policies by the Blood Banks and Blood Transfusion Services. Contrary to this hypothesis, we believe that Blood Banks and Blood Transfusion Services should continue their natural responsibility in the choice of filters and filtration procedures, in maintaining a centralized facility for the management of quality control data and in providing consultation on leucoreduction and feed-back of the results achieved to the clinicians. In particular, end users of leucoreduced blood components should be informed on the effectiveness of leucoreduction in achieving the desired prevention of blood transfusion complications. This is feasible by the circulation through the Transfusion Committee of quality indicators of leucoreduction policies such as incidence of NHFTR, CMV transmission, HLA alloimmunization, refractoriness to random platelet support, etc., in pertinent patient categories.

Pre-storage *versus* post-storage white cell depletion

A large body of evidence supports the need for early depletion of leucocytes to prevent the infusion of white cell fragments derived from cell disintegration during storage ('up-front filtration') (Engelfriet et al. 1975, Blajchman et al. 1992, Ramos et al. 1994). However, leucoreduction should not be performed too early, in order to preserve the bactericidal capacity of integral polymorphonuclear phagocytes during the first hours after blood collection (Högman et al. 1991). A definitive balance of these two opposite requirements has not been determined. A non-biological factor involved in the final choice is related to practical aspects including the timing and location of blood donation sessions, and the organization of blood component preparation. In some countries blood drives take place in afternoon - early evening hours, which can make more practical to hold at 20-24°C whole blood units until the next morning, thus starting their processing 12-16 hours after blood donation. The exact definition of the ideal holding time interval between donation and blood component preparation needs further investigation.

The use of blood components stored for more than a few days for recipients requiring leucoreduced components should be discouraged, to prevent the aforementioned risk of infusing leucocyte fragments that could theoretically cause HLA alloimmunization or cytokines released by leucocytes. However, recent *in vitro* data support the opposite view of less importance for the white cell fragments in regard to HLA alloimmunization (Dzik et al. 1994).

The issue of storage is also relevant for a possibility that has been developed by Mincheff and coworkers (1993), who proposed that the initial transfusion of non-leucoreduced RBC stored for some weeks might make the recipient unable to become alloimmunized to HLA after subsequent challenges with blood components containing HLA-bearing cells. This possibility, which is supported by in vitro data (Opelz and Terasaki 1974), requires to be evaluated in clinical trials.

The possibility of storing leucoreduced blood components has been documented in a number of studies (Lovric et al. 1981, Davey et al. 1989, Bertolini et al. 1992). In addition, these studies show that early white cell removal prevents the development of some storage lesions in RBC and in PC (Andreu 1991). The clinical relevance of this prevention needs to be determined.

Perspectives for the near future

In spite of the limited number of established recommended indications to the use of leucoreduced blood components (Lane et al. 1992, The Royal College of Physicians 1993), it has been suggested that leucoreduction might become a generalized procedure for all blood components in the near future. Notwithstanding the lack of complete scientific evidence on the cost-effectiveness of this policy, several Institutions use routine leucoreduction to prevent anti-HLA alloimmunization in leukaemic recipients of RBC and platelets. In a recent survey circulated to 32 Italian haematology units of the GIMEMA group (Gruppo Italiano Malattie Ematologiche Maligne dell'Adulto) participating in a clinical trial on platelet transfusion in leukaemia, 21 (66%) reported the routine use of leucoreduced blood components in their patients (GIMEMA, unpublished).

In addition, the possibility that leucoreduction is applied in some hospitals notwithstanding the lack of precise recommendations and clear evidence of its cost-effectiveness is suggested by the presence in the literature of articles and editorials discussing patient categories in whom routine leucoreduction of blood components does not seem to be indicated with the present level of knowledge.

This aspect is of special concern with reference to leucoreduction if the high cost of filters is considered. In this regard, efforts are being developed in several countries through the adoption of guidelines and protocols that should allow the maintenance of good levels of clinical practice at acceptable cost notwithstanding the continuous growth of request for expensive technology by patients and their lawyers.

In conclusion, clinical experience with leucoreduced blood components is far from having clarified all aspects of this important technology. Notwithstanding the great improvements recently achieved in regard to the efficacy of filters and filtration procedures, further work is required by the blood transfusion community to provide definitive answers to several critical issues. In our opinion, the most important include: maximum acceptable white cell levels in different conditions, clinical indications and quality control procedures.

References

Akahoshi M., Takanashi M., Masuda M., Yamashita H., Hidano A., Hasegawa K., Kasajima T., Shimizu M., Motoji T., Oshimi K., Mizoguchi H. (1992) A case of transfusion-associated graft-versus-host disease not prevented by white cell-reduction filters, *Transfusion* 32: 169-172.

Al E.L.M., Visser S.C.E., Broersen S.M., Stienstra S., Huisman J.G. (1993) Reduction of HTLV-infected cells in blood by leukocyte filtration, *Ann. Hematol.* 67: 295-300.

Anderson K.C., Goodnough L.T., Sayers M., Pisciotto P.T., Kurtz S.R., Lane T.A., Anderson C.S., Silberstein L.E. (1991) Variation in blood component irradiation practice: implications for prevention of transfusion-associated graft-versus-host disease, *Blood* 77: 2096-2102.

Andreu G., Dewailly J., Leberre C., Quarre M.C., Bidet M.L., Tardivel R., Devers L., Lam Y., Soreau E., Boccaccio C., Piard N., Bidet J.M., Genetet B., Fauchet R. (1988) Prevention of HLA immunization with leukocyte-poor packed red cells and platelet concentrates obtained by filtration, *Blood* 72: 964-969.

Andreu G. (1991) Early leukocyte depletion of cellular blood components reduces red blood cell and platelet storage lesions, *Sem. Hematol.* 28 (suppl 5): 22-25.

Andreu G., Boccaccio C., Klaren J., Lecrubier C., Pirenne F., Garcia I., Baudard M., Devers L., Fournel J.J. (1992) The role of UV radiation in the prevention of human leukocyte antigen alloimmunization, *Transf. Med. Rev.* 6: 212-224.

Anonymous (1992) Quality control approaches to leukocyte removal technology, *Clinical Lab. Letter* 13: 163-164.

Anonymous (1994) Catching the wave of progress in Miami: COBE Spectra User's Group, *Hémasphere* 7: 2-3.

Bertolini F., Rebulla P., Marangoni F., Sirchia G. (1992) Platelet concentrates stored in synthetic medium after filtration, *Vox Sang.* 62: 82-86.

Blajchman M.A., Bardossy L., Carmen R.A., Goldman M., Heddle N.M., Singal D.P. (1992) An animal model of allogeneic donor platelet refractoriness: the effect of pre-storage leukodepletion, *Blood* 79: 1371-1375.

Blumberg N., Heal J.M. (1987) Transfusion and host defenses against cancer recurrence and infection, *Transfusion* 29: 236-245.

Blumberg N., Triulzi D.J., Heal J.M. (1990) Transfusion-induced immunomodulation and its clinical consequences, *Transf. Med. Rev.* 4 (suppl. 1): 24-35.

Bowden R.A., Slichter S.J., Sayers M.H., Mori M., Cays M.J., Meyers J.D. (1991) Use of leukocyte-depleted platelets and cytomegalovirus-seronegative red blood cells for prevention of primary cytomegalovirus infection after marrow transplant, *Blood* 78: 246-250.

Brittingham T.E., Chaplin H. (1957) Febrile transfusion reactions caused by sensitivity to donor leukocytes and platelets, *JAMA* 167: 819-825.

Brubaker D.B. (1990) Clinical significance of white cell antibodies in febrile nonhemolytic transfusion reactions, *Transfusion* 30: 733-737.

Bruisten S.M., Tersmette M., Wester M.R., Vos A.H.V., Koppelman M.H.G.M., Huisman J.G. (1990) Efficiency of white cell filtration and freeze-thaw procedure for removal of HIV-infected cells from blood, *Transfusion* 30: 833-837.

Cao A., Gabutti V., Masera G., Modell B., Sirchia G., Vullo C. (1992) *Management Protocol for the Treatment of Thalassemia Patients*, Cooley's Anemia Foundation, New York.

Chambers L.A., Kruskall M.S., Pacini D.G., Donovan L.M. (1990) Febrile reactions after platelet transfusion: the effect of single versus multiple donors, *Transfusion* 30: 219-221.

Claas F.H.J., Smeenk R.J.T., Smidt R., Van Steenbrugge G.J., Eernisse J.G. (1981) Allo-immunization against the MHC antigens after platelet transfusion is due to contaminating leucocytes in the platelet suspension, *Exp. Hematol.* 9: 84-89.

Council of Europe (1992) *Guide to the Preparation, Use and Quality Assurance of Blood Components*, Council of Europe Press, Strasbourg.

Dacie J.V., Lewis S.M. (1991) *Practical Haematology* (7th ed.), Churchill Livingstone, Edinburgh.

Davey R.J., Carmen R.A., Simon T.L., Nelson E.J., Leng B.S., Chong C., Garcez R.B., Sohmer P.R. (1989) Preparation of white cell-depleted red cells for 42-day storage using an integral in-line filter, *Transfusion* 29: 496-499.

De Graan Hentzen Y.C.E., Gratama J.W., Mudde G.C., Verdonk L.F., Houbiers J.G.A., Brand A., Sebens F.W., Van Loon A.M., The T.H., Willemze T., De Gast G.C. (1989) Prevention of primary cytomegalovirus infection in patients with hematologic malignancies by intensive white cell depletion of blood products, *Transfusion* 29: 757-60.

Décary F., Ferner P., Giavedoni L., Hartman A., Howie R., Kalovsky E., Laschinger C., Malette M., Martyres A., Mervart H., Naylor D.H., St Rose J.E.M., Shepherd F.A., Tibensky D. (1984) An investigation of nonhemolytic transfusion reactions, *Vox Sang.* 46: 277-285.

Dumont L.J. (1991) Sampling errors and the precision associated with counting very low numbers of white cells in blood components, *Transfusion* 31: 428-432.

Dzik W.H. (1992) Is the febrile response to transfusion due to donor or recipient cytokine? (letter), *Transfusion* 32: 594.

Dzik S., Szuflad P., Eaves S. (1994) HLA antigens on leukocyte fragments and plasma proteins: prestorage leukoreduction by filtration, *Vox Sang.* 66: 104-111.

Eisenfeld L., Silver H., McLaughlin J., Klevjer-Anderson P., Mayo D., Anderson J., Herson V., Krause P., Savidakis J., Lazar A., Rosenkrantz T., Pisciotto P. (1992) Prevention of transfusion-associated cytomegalovirus infection in neonatal patients by the removal of white cells from blood, *Transfusion* 32: 205-209.

Engelfriet C.P., Diepenhorst P., Van den Giessen M., Von Riesz E. (1975) Removal of leucocytes from whole blood and erythrocyte suspensions by filtration through cotton wool. IV. Immunization studies in rabbits, *Vox Sang.* 28: 81-89.

Fisher M., Chapman J.R., Ting A., Morris P.J. (1985) Alloimmunisation to HLA antigens following transfusion with leucocyte-poor and purified platelet suspensions, *Vox Sang.* 49: 331-335.

Gilbert G.L., Hayes K., Hudson I.L., James J. and the Neonatal Cytomegalovirus Infection Study Group (1989) Prevention of transfusion-acquired cytomegalovirus infection in infants by blood filtration to remove leucocytes, *Lancet* 1: 1228-1231.

Goodnough T.L., Riddell J.I.V., Lazarus H., Chafel T.L., Prince G., Hendrix D., Yomtovian R. (1993) Prevalence of platelet transfusion reactions before and after implementation of leukocyte-depleted platelet concentrates by filtration, *Vox Sang.* 65: 103-107.

Heim M.U., Munker R., Sauer H., Wolf-Hornung B., Knabe H., Holler E., Böck M., Mempel W. (1991) Graft-versus-host Krankheit (GvH) mit letalem Ausgang nach der Gabe von gefilteren Erythrozytenkonzentraten (EK) (abstract), *Infusionstherapie* 18 (suppl. 2): 8-9.

Högman C.F., Gong J., Eriksson L., Hambraeus A., Johansson C.S. (1991) White cells protect donor blood against bacterial contamination, *Transfusion* 31: 612-626.

International Forum (1992) Should all platelet concentrates issued be leukocyte-poor?, *Vox Sang.* 62: 57-64.

Kiessling A.A., Crowell R.C., Brettler D., Forsberg A. (1993) Human immunodeficiency virus detection and differential leukocyte counts are accurate and safer with formaldehyde-fixed blood, *Blood* 81: 864-865.

Lamberson H.V., Dock N.L. (1992) Prevention of transfusion-transmitted cytomegalovirus infection, *Transfusion* 32: 196-198.

Lane T.A., Anderson K.C., Goodnough L.T., Kurtz S., Moroff G., Pisciotto P.T., Sayers M., Silberstein L.E. (1992) Leukocyte reduction in blood component therapy, *Ann. Int. Med.* 117: 151-162.

Lovric V.A., Schuller M., Raftos J., Wisdom L. (1981) Filtered microaggregate-free erythrocyte concentrates with 35-day shelf life, *Vox Sang.* 41: 6-10.

Mangano M.M., Chambers C.A., Kruskall M.S. (1991) Limited efficacy of leukopoor platelets for prevention of febrile transfusion reactions, *Am. J. Clin. Pathol.* 95: 733-738.

Masse M., Andreu G., Angue M., Babault C., Beaujean F., Bidet M.L., Boudart D., Calot J.P., Cotte C., Follea G., Gerota J., Hau F., Hurel C., Legrand E., Marchesseau B., Nasr O., Robert F., Royer D., Schooneman F., Tardivel R., Vidal M. (1992) A multicenter study on the efficiency of white cell reduction by filtration of red cells, *Transfusion* 32: 792-797.

Mincheff M.S., Meryman H.T., Kapoor V., Alsop P., Wötzel M. (1993) Blood transfusion and immunomodulation: a possible mechanism, *Vox Sang.* 65: 18-24.

Mintz P.D. (1991) Febrile reactions to platelet transfusions, *Am. J. Clin. Pathol.* 95: 609-611.

Moroff G., Luban N.L.C. (1992) Prevention of transfusion-associated graft-versus-host disease, *Transfusion* 32: 102-103.

Moroff G., Eich J., Dabay M. (1994) Validation of use of the Nageotte hemocytometer to count low levels of white cells in white cell-reduced platelet components, *Transfusion* 34: 35-38.

Muylle L., Joos M., Wouters E., De Bock R., Peetermans M.E. (1993) Increased tumor necrosis factor α (TNFα), interleukin 1, and interleukin 6 (IL-6) levels in the plasma of stored platelet concentrates: relationship between TNFα and IL-6 levels and febrile transfusion reactions, *Transfusion* 33: 195-199.

Muylle L., Peetermans M.E. (1994) Effect of prestorage leukocyte removal on the cytokine levels in stored platelet concentrates, *Vox Sang* 66: 14-17.

Nathanson S.D., Tilley B.C., Schultz L., Smith R.F. (1985) Perioperative allogeneic blood transfusions: survival in patients with resected carcinomas of the colon and rectum, *Arch. Surg.* 120: 734-738.

Nowak M.M., Ponsky J.L. (1984) Blood transfusion and disease-free survival in carcinoma of the breast, *J. Surg. Oncol.* 27: 124-130.

Okochi K., Sato H. (1986) Transmission of adult T-cell leukemia virus (HTLV-1) through blood transfusion and its prevention, *AIDS Res.* 2 (suppl): 157-161.

Oksanen K., Kekomäki R., Ruutu T., Koskimies S., Myllylä G. (1991) Prevention of alloimmunization in patients with acute leukemia by use of white cell-reduced blood components - a randomized trial, *Transfusion* 31: 588-94.

Opelz G., Terasaki P.I. (1974) Lymphocyte antigenicity loss with retention of responsiveness, *Science* 184: 464-466.

Perkins H.A., Payne R., Ferguson J., Wood M. (1966) Nonhemolytic febrile transfusion reactions. Quantitative effects of blood components with emphasis on isoantigenic incompatibility of leukocytes, *Vox Sang.* 11: 578-600.

Pietersz R.N.I., Steneker I., Reesink H.W., Dekker W.J.A., Al E.J.M., Huisman J.G., Biewenga J. (1992) Comparison of five different filters for the removal of leukocytes from red cell concentrates, *Vox Sang.* 62: 76-81.

Prati D., Capelli C., Bosoni P., Rebulla P. (1994) An improved method for white cell counting in white cell depleted red blood cells, *Transfusion* 34 (in press).

Ramos R.R., Curtis B.R., Duffy B.F., Chaplin H. (1994) Low retention of white cell fragments by polyester fiber white cell-reduction platelet filters, *Transfusion* 34: 31-34.

Rawal B.D., Busch M.P., Endow R., Garcia-de-Lomas J., Perkins H.A., Schwadron R., Vyas G.N. (1989) Reduction of human immunodeficiency virus-infected cells from donor blood by leukocyte filtration, *Transfusion* 29: 460-462.

Rebulla P., Porretti L., Bertolini F., Marangoni F., Prati D., Smacchia C., Pappalettera M., Parravicini A., Sirchia G. (1993) White cell reduced red blood cells prepared by filtration: a critical evaluation of current filters and methods for counting residual white cells, *Transfusion* 33: 128-133.

Rebulla P., Dzik W.H. (1994) Multicenter evaluation of methods for counting residual white cells in leukocyte-depleted red blood cells, *Vox Sang.* 66: 25-32.

Riccardi D., Raspollini E., Rossini G., Porretti L., Cordini S., Parravicini A., Rebulla P., Sirchia G. (1993) Reactions reported to red blood cells without buffy-coat and to platelet concentrates prepared from buffy-coats, *Transfusion* 33 (Suppl): 42s.

Sanders M.R., Graeber J.E. (1990) Posttransfusion graft-versus-host disease in infancy, *J. Pediatr.* 117: 159-163.

Schiffer C.A. (1991) Prevention of alloimmunization against platelets, *Blood* 77: 1-4.

Sintnicolaas K., Van Putten W.L.J. (1993) Comparison of four filters for leukocyte depletion of single donor plateletpheresis products, *Transfus. Sci.* 14: 211-215.

Sirchia G., Rebulla P., Mascaretti L., Greppi N., Andreis C., Rivolta S., Parravicini A. (1986) The clinical importance of leukocyte depletion in regular erythrocyte transfusions, *Vox Sang.* 51 (suppl. 1): 2-8.

Sirchia G., Parravicini A., Rebulla P. (1988) Leucocyte-depleted blood components, in: Cash J.D. (ed.) *Progress in Transfusion Medicine*, Vol 3, Churchill Livingstone, Edinburgh, pp. 87-109.

Sirchia G., Wenz B., Rebulla P., Parravicini A., Carnelli V., Bertolini F. (1990) Removal of white cells by transfusion through a new filter, *Transfusion* 30: 30-33.

Sirchia G., Rebulla P., Parravicini A., Marangoni F., Cortelezzi A., Stefania A. (1994) Quality control of red cell filtration at the patient's bedside, *Transfusion* 34: 26-30.

Stack G., Snyder E.L. (1994) Cytokine generation in stored platelet concentrates, *Transfusion* 34: 20-25.

Standards Committee (1993) Changes in the standards, *News Briefs* 15: 8-13.

Tegtmeier G.E. (1989) Posttransfusion cytomegalovirus infections, *Arch. Pathol. Lab. Med.* 13: 236-245.

Thaler M., Shamiss A., Orgad S., Huszar M., Nussinovitch N., Meisel S., Gazit E., Lavee J., Smolinsky A. (1989) The role of blood from HLA-homozygous donors in fatal transfusion-associated graft-versus-host disease after open-heart surgery, *NEJM* 321: 25-28.

The Royal College of Physicians of Edinburgh (1993) *Consensus Conference. Leucocyte Depletion of Blood and Blood Components*, Edinburgh.

Triulzi D.J., Vanek K., Ryan D.H., Blumberg N. (1992) A clinical and immunologic study of blood transfusion and postoperative bacterial infection in spinal surgery, *Transfusion* 32: 517-524.

Verdonk L.F., Middeldorp J.M., Kreeft H.A.G., Hauw The T., Hekker A., De Gast G.C. (1985) Primary cytomegalovirus infection and its prevention after autologous bone marrow transplantation, *Transplant.* 39: 455-457.

Voogt P.J., Van de Velde C.J., Brand A., Hermans J., Stijnen T., Bloem R., Leer J.W., Zwaveling A., Van Rood J.J. (1987) Perioperative blood transfusion and cancer prognosis: different effects of blood transfusion on prognosis of colon and breast cancer patients, *Cancer* 59: 836-843.

Vos J.J.E., Schoen C., Prins H.K., Von dem Borne A.E.G.Kr., Huisman J.G. (1987) Use of radioimmunoassay detecting the platelet glycoprotein IIb-IIIa complex, *Vox Sang.* 53: 23-25.

Walker R.H. (ed.) (1993) *Technical Manual* (11th ed.), American Association of Blood Banks, Bethesda, MD.

Wenz B. (1992) Leukocyte depletion filters should be used with apheresis platelets, *J. Clin. Apheresis.* 7: 149-150.

Wester M.R., Prins H.K., Huisman J.G. (1990) A new radioimmunoassay for the detection of small amounts of white cells and platelets in red cell concentrates: implications for blood transfusion, *Transfusion* 30: 117-125.

Widmann F.K. (ed.) (1985) *Technical Manual* (9th ed.), American Association of Blood Banks, Arlington, VA.

Widmann F.K. (ed.) (1993) *Standards for Blood Banks and Transfusion Services* (15th ed.), American Association of Blood Banks, Bethesda, MD.

Zurlo M.G., De Stefano P., Borgna Pignatti C., Di Palma A., Piga A., Melevendi C., Di Gregorio F., Burattini M.G., Terzoli S. (1989) Survival and causes of death in thalassaemia major, *Lancet* 2: 27-30.

Measurement of Low Numbers of Leucocytes
How should it be done?

9 | M. Masse

The recent development of filters used for leucocyte (WBC) reduction, together with the evolution of apheresis procedures have made it possible to obtain cell suspensions (red blood cells and platelet suspensions) which contain less and less contaminating leucocytes. More and more ambitious clinical objectives related to the prevention of HLA alloimmunization, virus transmission or bacterial infection, justify the use of leucocyte-depleted blood products.

To satisfy such clinical requirements, the availability of reliable, and sensitive counting techniques appears necessary for the determination of low numbers of leucocytes. The current quality requirement states a limit of residual leucocytes which must not exceed $1x10^6$ (4 WBC/μL), and even $1x10^5$ WBC (2 WBC/μL) in some clinical protocols (Andreu et al. 1993), per unit of transfused blood product.

Various techniques have been developed and reported. The validation of some of them, based on flow cytometry (FC) or using a Nageotte chamber (NC) has been the object of multicenter studies (Rebulla et al. 1994, Masse et al. 1991): they are now commonly used for the routine quality control of WBC-depleted blood products (Lambrey et al. 1993, Moroff et al. 1994, Rebulla et al. 1993). Current research aims at further increasing the sensitivity of these counting methods, so as to assess the actual performance (generally expressed in log depletion [Sadoff et al. 1991, Wenz et al. 1991]) of novel filtration materials and thus determine new clinical objectives that are beneficial to transfused patients. Some methods, such as quantitative polymerase chain reaction (PCR), the cytospin technique, cell sorting with immunomagnetic beads, cytometric methods applied to a filtrating membrane are still at their experimental stage.

Some of them, like PCR are in the process of being validated (Takahashi et al. 1993, Lee et al. 1993) and need to be simplified in order to be more widely used. Counting on a Nageotte chamber is currently recognized worldwide as the reference method (Rebulla et al. 1994).

Criteria to be considered in the choice of a counting method

Among the criteria which are likely to impact on the choice of a counting method, reliability, precison, reproducibility are essential, but rapidity, simplicity and low cost are also elements that must be taken into account (Dzik 1991). In order to be considered as efficient, a method must be generalized to all of the laboratories and be familiar to technologists. Interlaboratory sample exchanges and training periods organized for technologists from various laboratories is a further step towards a better standardization.

Thus, the work carried out on the occasion of multicenter studies has made it possible to determine limits of precision, which depend on the counting method (by flow cytometry or with a Nageotte chamber) and above all on the WBC-concentration range to be measured. The sensitivity threshold is another important criterion to be considered in the choice of a counting method. Thus, different counting methods must be used for a concentration of approximately 0.01 WBC/μL and one of 10 WBC/μL, given that the coefficients of variation (CV%) for one method generally differ when sensitivity varies by a 10^3 factor (Rebulla et al. 1993).

The theoretical sensitivity limit of a counting method, which is related to its detection limit, in other terms to the enumeration or quantitation of an event (1 WBC) must not be separated from its limit of precision, which is equivalent to the reading of about 10 events (WBCs) in a counting chamber (Masse et al. 1992): detection limit = sensitivity limit x10.

The sensitivity limits (WBC/μL) of various counting methods, are illustrated hereby (see Figure 1).

Figure 1 *Comparative sensitivity limits of various counting methods*

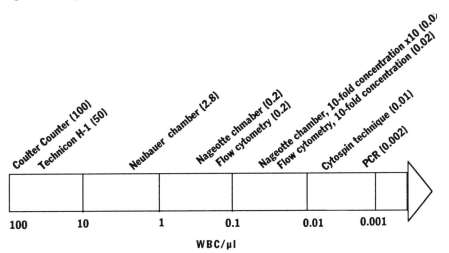

The limit of precision is related to two parameters: the volume and concentration of the sample to be assayed (Dumont 1991). It is divided by 2 when the volume is doubled. In addition, several studies have demonstrated a substantial improvement in the coefficient of variation following concentration of the sample by centrifugation (5-, 10- or 20-fold) (Rebulla et al. 1994, Lambrey et al. 1993, Takahashi et al. 1993, Masse et al. 1992). The sample volume must be compatible with the future use in transfusion of the controlled blood product. Thus, no method leading to the destruction of the product can be adopted in routine use, even if the quality control procedures for WBC-reduced blood components do not apply to all of the products, but only to a small proportion (1 to 5%). Therefore, if these controls are to be representative of the quality level of filtration, it is essential to define a standardized filtration procedure beforehand, ensure its correct application and also respect strict rules when sampling (such as performing at least a triple stripping on a tube which is at least 20 cm in length, together with a storage time which does not exceed 24 hours before counting).

All of these precautions should orientate one's choice towards a counting method which has been effectively validated.

Validation protocol

In addition to the document that provides a detailed description of the counting procedure they use, technicians in the control laboratory must constitute a validation document which guarantees that results are in conformance with acceptability criteria. An example of such a document is provided in the following diagram (see Figure 2).

Figure 2 *Flow diagram of a validation procedure*

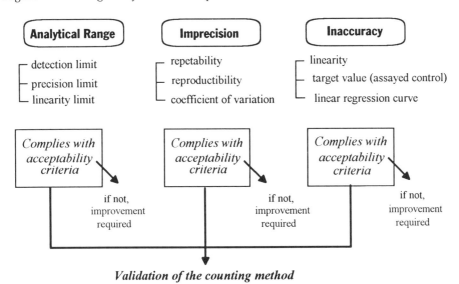

Validation of the counting method

A validation procedure generally includes the following steps:

- Assessment of the analytical range includes assessing the detection limit (sensitivity threshold) and the linearity limit. In other words, this involves determining the concentration range over which the technique can be used (e.g.,

between 0.1 and 10 WBC/μL with FC or NC). A range, including 3 to 4 samples with a known concentration, is performed in the linearity range under control.
- Assessment of precision via repeatability and reproducibility assays. A 20 to 30% coefficient of variation is generally admitted.
- Assessment of accuracy and plotting of a linear regression curve between observed and expected values, in the previously defined linearity range.
- Comparison with a reference method, if it does exist, and determination of a coefficient of correlation.

The multicenter evaluation of two types of methods (NC and FC) has been the object of workshops organized by the BEST and PSL groups, in which validation protocols have been established for them. These methods should obviously be preferred when measuring WBC concentrations over the 0.1 to 10 WBC/μL range.

Validated counting methods

The flow cytometric (FC) method

This method involves nuclear staining of cell suspensions with a DNA/RNA fluorophore: propidium iodide. Flow cytometry is an extremely powerful research tool for the multiparameter analysis of rare events, notably for the identification of WBC subpopulations, as has been demonstrated by B. Wenz et al. (1991) and E. Al et al. (1991).

Under the action of a vector fluid, the fluorescent dye-stained cells are first excited by an incident laser beam and subsequently enumerated. This method requires extreme care during calibration procedures, notably when setting analytic gates - the areas where signals are detected and must be distinguished from background noise and cell debris). There is no standard calibration nor is there any calibration that could be used from one laboratory to another. Flow cytometry involves a lengthy procedure. The apparatuses can analyze 1 μL of sample per second, and if the operator is patient, it can analyze over 1 mL. This constitutes an advantage for this method, since, as was demonstrated by Dumont (1991), the accuracy of any counting methods is closely linked to the volume of the sample under analysis.

Various types of apparatuses can be used for the quantitation of residual WBCs in filtered red blood cell or platelet suspensions: Ortho Cytoron (Orthodiagnostic System), FACScan (Becton Dickinson) and Epics Profile II (Coulter Electronics). The sample to be counted is generally diluted 1:10 and the volume of the counted sample is approximately 1 mL.

With the Ortho Cytoron apparatus, Takahashi et al. (1993) obtained excellent correlation coefficients (r=0.999) as compared to a Nageotte hemocytometer, for concentrations ranging from 0.4 to 40 WBC/μL, on red blood cell (RBC) or platelet concentrates (PC).

FACScan and Epics apparatuses were tested on RBC concentrates during the first multicenter workshop held by the international BEST group (Rebulla et al. 1994). The aim was to determine the lower detection limit for FC and NC. Several laboratories followed a common protocol and tested these methods using calibration samples of 10^{-3} and 10^3 cells/μL, prepared by dilution of BC-depleted RBCs with red blood cells filtered three times. Depending on the equipment used, the volume aspirated varied from 0.5 to 1.5 mL, with the dilution factor ranging from 11 to 16. The study demonstrated a low interlaboratory variability, acceptable up to the limit of 0.1 WBC/μL. A similar limit of precision was reached with the Cytoron. The first results of this method suggest the FC method should be reserved to evaluate the performances of novel filtering material (3 to 5 $\log_{10}$ depletion) rather than be used for routine quality control.

The Nageotte hemocytometer
It is by far the most widely used method. Its advantage lies in its simplicity, low cost and large volume in comparison with other hemocytometers (Neubauer: 1.5 μL, Bürker: 0.8 μL, Mallassez: 1 μL, Fuchs Rosenthal: 3.2 μL, Nageotte: 50 μL).

With this method, WBC counting is performed under a microscope (x20 magnification), following RBC lysis and 1:10 dilution of the sample with either Plaxan or Türk's solution.

Either 50 or 10 μL of this sample are transferred to the Nageotte chamber equipped with one or two 40-rectangle counting grids and an underside metal coating (special Brightlight version). After a sedimentation time of about 15 minutes, readings are performed by 1 or 2 operators in less than 10 min. WBC concentration is expressed as:

$$C = \frac{N}{V \times K}$$

C = concentration (WBC/μL)
N = number of WBCs seen in the chamber
V = volume of the chamber (50 or 100 μL)
K = dilution factor (here 1:10)

Sensitivity, linearity range, precision, accuracy and correlation curve have been the object of several studies and publications, so that counting on a Nageotte hemocyometer is now a reference method (BEST/PSL), with a CV lower than 25% for concentrations higher than 2.5 WBC/μL. Its analytical range is generally admitted to be situated between 0.5×10^6 and 5×10^6 WBC/unit. This method is quite satisfactory for the routine quality control of RBC or platelet concentrates that have been filtered with 3 $\log_{10}$ depletion filters (such as Pall, BPF4, LRF6, Sepacell RS200, PLS5 for instance). The goal is to ensure that the rate of blood components which do not comply with a previously defined quality objective (WBC > 1×10^6 per unit) is minimum and even nought. And in this case, determining the actual performance of the filter or the number of residual WBCs in the transfused unit is not the essential concern. For their determination, either the modified Nageotte technique or other more sophisticated methods should be privileged.

Modified counting methods with the Nageotte chamber

The modification made in the counting method aims primarily at improving sensitivity, this can be increased by modifying the sample volume and the dilution factor. Several protocols have been suggested, some of which have already been the object of multicenter studies (BEST working party).

Validated protocol, as developed by Dzik (1991)
A mixture of Türk's solution and Zap-oglobin - a commercial RBC lysing agent (Coulter Diagnostics) - is used to dilute and lyse 100 μL of the RBC sample diluted 1:5. The sensitivity is thus reduced by half (1 counted WBC = 0.1 WBC/μL).

Validated protocol, as developed by Masse (Rebulla et al. 1994, Masse et al. 1992)
One or 2 mL of the initial sample are diluted 1:10, using Plaxan solution - an RBC lysing solution (Fiers-Belgium) - and adjusted to 1 mL, prior to reading. Sensitivity is thus reduced 10- or 20-fold (it is interesting to note that this protocol is also applicable to platelet suspensions, provided Plaxan is replaced by 3% acetic acid). Over the 0.1 to 5 WBC/μL range, precision is markedly higher than in the previous protocols. Moreover, given the analytical range thus reached (0.5×10^4 - 0.5×10^5 WBC per unit), this protocol should be reserved to the validation of current filters (BPF4, RS200) or to the evaluation of novel, more efficient filters (e.g., 6 $\log_{10}$ depletion filters).

Protocol being validated, as developed by Prati (internal communication, BEST group, unpublished)
In this protocol, a 10-mL RBC suspension is lysed and diluted 1:5 with 3% paraformaldehyde and adjusted to 0.5 mL with Plaxan solution following centrifugation. Linearity over the 0.005-5 WBC/μL concentration range appears quite satisfactory, so does precision. This protocol could be used to evaluate high-performance filters (6 $\log_{10}$ depletion).

Table 1 *Characteristics of various counting protocols using a Nageotte hemocytometer*

Dilution factor	Sample volume	Theoretical sensitivity	Precision limit	Analytical range	Leucocyte detection threshold
Protocol	mL	WBC/μL	WBC/μL	WBC/μL	WBC/unit
0.1 (BEST/PSL)	0.1	0.2	2	2-10	6×10^5
0.2 (BEST/Dzik)	0.1	0.1	1	1-5	3×10^5
1 (BEST/Masse)	1	0.02	0.2	0.2-1	6×10^4
2 (Masse)	2	0.01	0.1	0.1-1	3×10^4
20 (Prati)	10	0.001	0.01	0.01-0.1	3×10^3

The Table 1 is a summary of the characteristics and analytical ranges of these various protocols using a Nageotte hemocytometer.

High sensitivity counting methods

The cytospin technique
This method has been described by two authors. Takahashi et al. (1993) determined the conditions required for the concentration and cytocentrifugation on a glass slide of a 5-mL sample of platelet or RBC concentrate. Between his hands, this technique was 10-fold more sensitive than the flow cytometric method (0.01 WBC/μL). The correlation curve comparing the hemocytometer and cytospin methods was however not very satisfactory.

Sadoff et al. (1991), as part of experiments carried out on novel filters (6 $\log_{10}$ depletion) applied the cytospin technique to mononuclear cells which had been isolated by Ficoll Hypaque gradient centrifugation. This technique is destructive: 300 to 350 mL of suspension are required. Its sensitivity was assessed as being 0.003 WBC/μL.

To date, complete validation cannot be expected. This technique should be left aside (it is not very reliable, not very reproducible and destructive) and replaced by a more sensitive technique, like PCR, on which high hopes are placed.

Quantitative Polymerase Chain Reaction (PCR)
Measurement of very low numbers of nucleated cells can be done using molecular biology methods. PCR allows in vitro selective amplification of DNA sequences which would otherwise be undetectable with conventional methods. This technique has been used on 0.5- to 1-mL samples of WBC-reduced red cells. First RBC lysis of the sample is performed (a critical step, since free hemoglobin may interfere with the assay) and DNA is extracted from the cell nucleus (approximately 6 g per nucleus), a DNA gene is chosen as a target for several amplification cycles. The amplification product, analyzed by electrophoresis on agarose gel (Southern Blot) is thus proportional to the initial number of nucleated cells.

Takahashi et al. (1993) chose to amplify Beta Globin gene, as it is well characterized and its primers are commercially available.

Lee et al. (1993) chose HLA DQ-alpha gene, which is also well characterized and already used for the DNA amplification of HIV-infected cells (Rawal et al. 1990).

Each of these studies showed a good correlation with the reference Nageotte method (r=0.97) over a common concentration range (0.1-10 WBC/μL) with however a 10- to 100-fold higher theoretical sensitivity (up to 0.002 cells/μL).

To date, quantitative PCR is certainly the most valuable method (labelling with a non radioisotope probe, reading on microplatelets, automated procedure) it must be developed to evaluate the performances of new-generation filters. It requires being perfected in order to be used on platelet suspensions.

Searching for new methods

Immunomagnetic bead sorting

This method has been adapted from bone marrow or peripheral blood stem cell purging methods. The sample is first incubated with magnetic beads (Dynal) coated with an anti-WBC monoclonal antibody, and leucocytes are then sorted and counted. No serious study has been undertaken yet and the sensitivity of the method is unknown.

Flow cytometry performed on a filtration membrane

This method which has been adapted for the counting of rare events in hematology, is now being investigated by the French PSL group and is the object of a multicenter validation protocol (unpublished data).

Following RBC lysis of a sample, dye-labelled nucleated cells with a cell nucleus-specific dye (propidium iodide) are filtered on a polycarbonate membrane, which has 1- to 3-μm calibrated pores. The cells thus isolated are identified by image analysis and quantified. Three blood transfusion centers applied a common experimental protocol (linearity, accuracy, repeatability, reproducibility) over a concentration range of 2 to 6 WBC/μL, this resulted in unsatisfactory validation. The method is currently insufficiently specific for the required sensitivity.

Conclusion

This broad inventory of counting methods used for the detemination of low numbers of leucocytes shows that perfect techniques do not exist.

The precision of results is related to the care exercised in counting, it is expressed by the coefficient of variation (20 to 30%). Compliance with a standardized protocol, implementation of inter- and intra-laboratory controls, frequent validation of counting procedures via assays performed over a reference range are all elements that are essential for the recognition and publication of a counting procedure.

Several important parameters must be taken into account for a good choice. First, the goal of quality control testing must be clearly stated: it is either routine quality control performed to check the quality of WBC-reduced blood products and determine the rate of units that do not comply with a critical threshold (e.g., 1x10^6 residual WBC/unit) or it is aimed at evaluating the performances of current or novel filters following a filtration procedure indicated by the manufacturer.

In the first instance, a simple, reliable and inexpensive technique should be chosen, such as counting a diluted sample on a Nageotte hemocytometer, or PCR.

In whatever situation, the selected method has to be standardized and validated, (linearity, precision, accuracy).

The development and perfection of counting methods for the determination of very low numbers of leucocytes, in conformance with good laboratory practices constitutes a quality objective which is beneficial to recipients of blood transfusion.

We should maybe concede that in this field, as in numerous other fields, nothing has been achieved yet, as the best is still to be achieved.

References

Al E.M.J. et al. (1991) A flow cyotometric method for determination of white cell subpopulations in filtered red cells, *Transfusion* 31: 835-842.

Andreu G. et al. (1993) Prevention of HLA alloimmunisation using UV-B irradiated platelet concentrates (PC): Results of a prospective randomized clinical trial (Abstract), *Transfusion* 33: S293.

Dumont L.J. (1991) Sampling errors and the precision associated with counting very low numbers of white cells in blood components, *Transfusion* 31: 428-432.

Dzik W.H. (1991) White cell-reduced blood components: Should we go with the flow?, *Transfusion* 31: 789-791.

Lambrey Y. et al. (1993) Description et validation d'une méthode cytofluorométrique d'estimation des leucocytes résiduels dans les concentrés globulaires déleucocytés, *Rev. Fr. Transfus. Hémobiol.* 36: 375-390.

Lee T.H. et al. (1993) Quantification of residual leukocytes in filtered blood components by polymerase chain reaction amplification of HLA DQ alpha DNA (Abstract), *Transfusion* 33: S35.

Masse M. et al. (1991) For the PSL working party of the French Society of Blood Transfusion. A multicenter study on the efficiency of white cell reduction by filtration of red cells, *Transfusion* 31: 792-797.

Masse M. et al. (1992) Validation of a simple method to count very low white cell concentration in filtered red cells or platelets, *Transfusion* 32: 564-571.

Moroff G. et al. (1994) Validation of use of the Nageotte hemocytometer to count low levels of white cells in white cell-reduced platelet concentrates, *Transfusion* 34: 35-38.

Rawal B.D. et al. (1990) Evaluation of leukocyte removal filters modelled by use of HIV-infected cells and DNA amplification, *Blood* 76: 2159-2161.

Rebulla P. et al. (1993) White cell-reduced red cells prepared by filtration:a critical evaluation of current filters and methods for counting residual white cells, *Transfusion* 33: 128-133.

Rebulla P. et al. (1994) For the biomedical excellence for safer transfusion (BEST) working party of the International Society of Blood Transfusion. Multicenter evalutation of methods for counting residual white cells in leukocyte-depleted red blood cells, *Vox Sang.* 66: 25-32.

Sadoff B.J. et al. (1991) Methods for measuring a 6 $\log_{10}$ white cell depletion in red cells, *Transfusion* 31: 150-155.

Takahashi T.A. et al. (1993) Comparison of highly sensitive methods used to count residual leukocytes in filtered red cell and platelet concentrates, in: Sekiguchi S. (ed.) *Clinical Application of Leukocyte Depletion*, Blackwell Scientific Publication, Oxford.

Wenz B. et al. (1991) A rare-event analysis model for quantifying white cells in white cell-depleted blood, *Transfusion* 31: 156-159.

Blood Transfusion - Cancer and Post Operative Infection

10 | N.R. Parrott

Introduction

The first human-to-human blood transfusion has been credited to James Blundell, and was given over 100 years ago. Early transfusion practice was fraught with danger and it was not until the discovery of blood groups by Landsteiner and Wiener in 1902 that transfusion gained some semblance of safety. The first blood bank was established in Chicago, and it was the advent of the Second World War that highlighted the need for large volumes of banked blood. Such a service is now a vital and integral part of routine clinical care.

Table 1 *Possible mechanisms of transfusion-associated immunosuppression or graft enhancement*

1. Selection of non-responders
2. Clonal deletion theory
3. Reduced MLR responsiveness
4. Altered macrophage activity
5. Changes in arachidonic acid metabolism
6. Reduced activity of Natural Killer cells
7. Non-specific immunosuppressive plasma proteins
8. Anti-idiotypic antibodies
9. Fc - receptor blocking antibodies
10. Altered cytokine activity (interleukin-2)

Whilst the dangers of mismatched transfusion were soon apparent, it was not until the work of Opelz (Opelz et al. 1973) in 1973 that the possibility of transfusion being immunosuppressive was considered. Opelz' observation that the multiple-transfused transplant recipient had improved allograft survival in comparison to the non-transfused recipient led to a wealth of clinical and laboratory research into this so called 'transfusion effect'. Most, if not all the clinical studies were other retrospective analyses of renal transplant outcome in relation to transfusion status. Virtually all of these seemed to confirm Opelz' findings, and many workers also identified profound immunological changes following blood transfusion (Kaplan et al. 1984, Nagarkatti et al. 1983, Borleffs et al. 1983, Waymack et al. 1986, Waymack et al. 1987, Stephan et al. 1988). This led many transplant units to adopt a mandatory pre-transplant transfusion protocol in renal allograft recipients. Such practices are still in place today, but it is interesting to note that such practices were so widely adopted in the absence of a methodologically (or statistically) sound prospective study. The possible mechanism(s) of the transfusion effect are outlined in Table 1.

Blood transfusion and cancer

It was a further decade before the possible association of blood transfusion with tumour recurrence was questioned by Burrows and Tartter (Burrows and Tartter 1982). In this retrospective study of patients with colorectal cancer, the authors reported a 5 year disease free survival of 84% in patients who did not receive blood transfusion, but a 51% disease free survival in patients receiving peri-operative blood transfusion. This initial observation opened the flood gates for other studies to examine the putative association of blood transfusion with cancer recurrence. Since then, there have been 30 studies in the literature that examine an association between transfusion and recurrence of colonic and rectal cancer. Whilst the numerical majority suggest that transfusion may be detrimental in patients with such tumours (Burrows et al. 1987, Blumberg et al. 1985, Beynon et al. 1989, Corman et al. 1986, Creasy et al. 1987, Foster et al. 1985, Francis and Judson 1987, Liewald et al. 1990, Parrott et al. 1986, Ross 1987, Voogt et al. 1987, Wobbes et al. 1989), there is also a significant number where no association is seen (Cheslyn et al. 1990, Frankish 1985, Jakobsen et al. 1990, Mecklin 1989, Nathanson et al. 1985, Ota et al. 1985, Quintiliani et al. 1991, Vente et al. 1989, Weiden et al. 1987). The total number of patients examined in all these studies is now around 6000, and yet the answer is still far from clear. The majority of these studies are retrospective, uncontrolled observational studies, in which there may be a large number of potentially confounding variables that may have resulted in a bias in the data. In a number of studies, the confounding effect of variables has been lessened by the use of multiple regression analysis. The latter technique allows the analysis of transfusion as an independent statistically significant predictor of recurrence or death from recurrence. Yet, why should there be such diversity of opinion in these studies? Firstly the studies vary greatly in number;- from less than 100 to over 900 patients. The statistical power of such studies is clearly variable. There is also considerable variability in the methodology in all of the studies. Some reflect the experience of centres with a particular interest in colorectal cancer, some are multi-centre (or multi-surgeon), some are single centre, and all have varying definitions of what constitutes 'peri-operative' transfusion. In the context of renal transplantation, the so called transfusion effect may be immunosuppressive even when blood was given many months (or years) prior to transplantation. In the colorectal cancer studies, none have examined the transfusion history of the patient more than a few weeks prior to colonic surgery. As almost all are retrospective studies, it is often difficult or impossible to determine what factor led to transfusion being required in the first place. As stated by Vamvakas and Moore in a recent review; 'peri-operative blood transfusion does not occur in a clinical vacuum, but is intertwined with many variables that are potentially related to tumour recurrence' (Vamvakas and Moore 1993). This is perhaps the most pertinent reason why such retrospective studies are difficult to interpret. Blood transfusion may be no more than a marker for the biologically more aggressive disease. In their in-depth and thoughtful review, Vamvakas and Moore have attempted to analyse all colorectal cancer studies with particular reference of confounding variables. They conclude that the current evidence is insufficient to warrant a change in transfusion practice, that the relative risk of cancer recurrence in transfused patients may be from 37-43%, and that this enhanced risk may be largely accounted for by confounding variables. They surmise that the *true* transfusion effect may be small, and amount to no more than 10-20% relative risk.

It would be difficult to agree with their conclusion however, and even if the risk of recurrence was reduced by only 10% by the avoidance of blood transfusion, then perhaps we should do so.

In another recent and extensive meta-analysis, Chung et al. (1993) suggested that their own review supported the hypothesis that transfusion may be associated with increased recurrence. They calculated the odds ratio of recurrence or cancer death as 1.80 and 1.76 respectively.

Blood transfusion and other cancers

All of the criticisms and comments about colorectal cancer apply equally to other forms of human cancer. Nevertheless, there are now few human cancers that have not been subject to scrutiny with respect to blood transfusion. These are reviewed only very briefly here.

Breast cancer

Not unnaturally, breast cancer has been examined in some detail, but the weight of data appears more in favour of there being no significant effect. So far as the author is aware, there has been no meta-analysis of breast cancer, but all are retrospective observational studies. There are 12 published studies of breast cancer and transfusion. Tartter's group suggested that transfusion may be detrimental to patients undergoing mastectomy with axillary clearance (Tartter et al. 1985). One hundred and sixty nine patients were studied, and 51% of the transfused patients were free of disease after 5 years. In the group that did not receive peri-operative blood, 65% were disease free. This 14% survival advantage was statistically significant, but these findings were not supported by the recent Danish Breast Cancer Co-operative group data (Eickhoff et al. 1991). Of the 12 studies in press, 9 suggest that there is no association of transfusion with cancer recurrence.

An important caveat must be added to the breast cancer studies. The biological behaviour of breast cancer is such that the analysis of recurrence may be inappropriate after 5 years. Meaningful data may require 10-20 year follow up.

Lung cancer
The published data with respect to lung tumour recurrence and transfusion is further confused by the differing histological sub-types. In those studies that have examined purely non-small-cell lung cancer (NSCLC), the evidence is divided. Two studies, from Tartter (Parrott 1993) and Little (Miholic et al. 1985) find transfusion to be detrimental, but those from Pastorino (Ottino et al. 1987) and Keiler do not do so (Murphy et al. 1991).

In the two further studies (Triulzi et al. 1992, Fernadez et al. 1992), a mixture of NSCLC and squamous tumours have been examined, and it has been suggested that blood transfusion may be associated with an adverse outcome.

Other tumours
The influence of transfusion has been questioned in a variety of other, less common human tumours including soft tissue sarcomas, prostatic, gastric, renal, genital, maxillofacial and metastatic liver cancer. In many of these studies, transfusion has been thought to have been detrimental to cancer free survival. These data are summarised in Table 2, and have been recently reviewed in more detail than here (Parrott 1993).

Table 2 *Summary of all published studies, irrespective of size or statistical analysis method*

Tumour	Significant effect	Non significant effect	Total
Colon and rectum	15	15	30
Breast	3	9	12
Stomach	3	2	5
Prostate	3	0	3
Kidney	1	2	3
Lung	4	2	6
Sarcoma	1	0	1
Liver metastases	2	0	2
Bone	1	0	1
Head & neck	3	1	4
Genitalia	1	3	4
	37 (52.1%)	34 (47.9%)	71 (100%)

Blood transfusion and infection

There are two contentious facets of the cancer/transfusion hypothesis; the role of the immune system in common human tumours and the diversity of behaviour of human malignancy. In septic states, these arguments are non-valid. Few could argue that the human immune system has a role against sepsis, and the presence of pus is easier to quantify objectively. Equally, there are no published studies that refute an association between transfusion and human sepsis.

In two early studies of patients undergoing cardiothoracic surgery (Miholic et al. 1985, Ottino et al. 1987), it was shown that blood transfusion was associated with a variety of septic complications. In the study by Miholic et al. (1985), 246 patients underwent valve replacement or coronary artery bypass grafting (CABG). By multivariate analysis, only blood transfusion, reoperation, and duration of cardiopulmonary bypass were associated with post-operative sepsis. In the study by Ottino, a multivariate analysis of 2,579 consecutive cardiac procedures was undertaken. Blood transfusion was one of six variables found to be associated with sternal wound infection on stepwise logistic regression analysis (Ottino et al. 1987). In 3 more recent studies, blood transfusion has been associated with enhanced post-operative sepsis in patients undergoing hip surgery (Murphy et al. 1991), spinal surgery (Triulzi et al. 1992), or a combination of hip, knee and spinal operations (Fernadez et al. 1992). In the study by Murphy et al. (1991), patients receiving allogeneic (homologous) blood had a 32% rate of proven sepsis, in comparison to those patients receiving autologous blood who had only a 3% incidence of post-operative infection.

Patients undergoing spinal surgery and receiving allogeneic transfusions (Triulzi et al. 1992) had longer operations and great blood loss than those receiving no blood, but also had a greater rate of infection (21% versus 4% respectively). In a variety of orthopaedic (Fernadez et al. 1992) or other surgical procedures (Mezrow et al. 1992), homologous blood, but not autologous was associated with a significantly enhanced risk of post-operative sepsis.

Tartter has also undertaken a prospective study of infectious complications in patients undergoing colorectal cancer surgery (Tartter 1988). In a series of 343 patients, 134 received transfusions, and 209 did not. The post-operative infection rates were 24.6 and 4.3% respectively ($p < 0.0001$). By multivariate analysis, transfusion was significantly associated with sepsis. Transfusion has also been associated with enhanced sepsis in patients with Crohns disease (Tartter et al. 1988) and following burn injury (Graves et al. 1989).

Risk reduction in transfusion

Many of the immediate adverse effects of blood transfusion are now well documented, and fortunately rare. However, whether blood transfusion is really putting our cancer patients at risk of recurrence is still unclear. The question could be answered by randomised prospective study, but so far only one such study has been published. The Rotterdam group randomised 424 patients to their prospective study of autologous versus autogeneic transfusion in patients undergoing surgery for colorectal cancer. 118 patients received allogeneic transfusions and only 59 received just autologous blood. Interestingly their study showed absolutely no difference in post-operative sepsis (25% and 29% respectively), and at a mean follow up of 42 months, disease free survival was 55% in each group (Busch et al. 1992).

One must sound a note of caution however. Whilst the Rotterdam study may appear to be compelling evidence against the hypothesis that transfusion of allogeneic blood may be detrimental, the same group have also published evidence to show that pre-deposit (or blood loss) is itself an immunosuppressive phenomenon, and the 'control' group (given pre-deposit blood) may also have been immunosuppressed for different reasons (Lawick van Pabst et al. 1988).

Whilst there are many other ways of avoiding allogeneic transfusion (Table 3), one of these has been studied by Jensen et al (Jensen et al. 1992). Patients undergoing elective colorectal surgery were randomised to receive 'unmodifed' allogeneic blood, or blood depleted of white cells by bedside filter. Post-operative sepsis occured in 2.2% of the non-transfused, in 2.1% of the patients with leucocyte depleted blood, and in 28% of those receiving whole blood (p < 0.01).

Table 3 *Techiques to eliminate the risk of allogeneic transfusion*

1.	Pre-deposit autotransfusion
2.	Isovolaemic haemodilution
3.	Peri-operative cell salvage
4.	Post-operative cell salvage
5.	White cell filtering
6.	Artificial blood subsitutes

Jensen's study represents intriguing possibilities for the future management of patients with allogeneic transfusion, and seems to suggest that it is the white cells in a transfusion that are responsible for the immunosuppression of transfusion. Clearly, there are many more questions that remain to be answered, but a prospective evaluation of the effect of leucocyte depleted blood on cancer recurrence may take 5 years to come.

References

Beynon J., Davies P.W., Billings P.J. et al. (1989) Perioperative blood transfusion increases the risk of recurrence in colorectal cancer, *Dis. Colon. Rectum* 32: 975-979.

Blumberg N., Agarwal M.M., Chuang C. (1985) Relation between recurrence of cancer of the colon and blood transfusion, *Br. Med. 3* 290: 1037-1039.

Borleffs J.C., Neuhaus P., Marquet R.L., Balner H. (1983) Blood transfusions and changes in humoral and cellular immune reactivity in rhesus monkeys. Possible predictive value for kidney allograft prognosis, *Transplantation* 35: 150-155.

Burrows L., Tartter P., Aufses A. (1987) Increased recurrence rates in perioperatively transfused colorectal malignancy patients, *Cancer Detect. Prev.* 10: 361-369.

Burrows L., Tartter P. (1982) Effect of blood transfusions on colonic malignancy recurrence rates, *Lancet* ii: 662.

Busch O.R.C., Hop W.C.J., Hoyuk van Papendrecht M.A.W., Marquet R.L., Jeekek J. (1992) Relationship between blood transfusion and recurrence of colorectal cancer: results from a prospective randomised study, *Eur. J. Surg. Oncol.* 18 (suppl. 2): 29.

Cheslyn-Curtis S., Fielding L.P., Hittinger R., Fry J.S., Phillips R.K. (1990) Large bowel cancer: the effect of perioperative blood transfusion on outcome, *Ann. Roy. Coll. Surg. Eng.* 72: 53-59.

Chung M., Steinmetz O.K., Gordon P.H. (1993) Perioperative blood transfusion and outcome after resection for colorectal carcinoma, *Br. J. Surg.* 80: 427-432.

Corman J., Arnoux R., Peloquin A., St-Louis G., Smeesters C., Giroux L. (1986) Blood transfusions and survival after colectomy for colorectal cancer, *Can. J. Surg.* 29: 325-329.

Creasy T.S., Veitch P.S., Bell P.R. (1987) A relationship between perioperative blood transfusion and recurrence of carcinoma of the sigmoid colon following potentially curative surgery, *Ann. R. Coll. Surg. Eng.* 69: 100-103.

Eickhoff J.H., Anderson J., Laybourne C. (1991) Perioperative blood transfusion does not promote recurrence and death after mastectomy for breast cancer, *Br. J. Surg.* 78: 1358.

Fernadez M.C., Gottlieb M., Menitove J.E. (1992) Blood transfusion and postoperative infection in orthopaedic patients, *Transfusion* 32: 318-322.

Foster R.S., Costanza M.C., Foster J.C., Wanner M.C., Foster C.B. (1985) Adverse relationship between blood transfusions and survival after colectomy for colon cancer, *Cancer* 55: 1195-1201.

Francis D.M., Judson R.T. (1987) Blood transfusion and recurrence of cancer of the colon and rectum, *Br. J. Surg.* 74: 26-30.

Frankish P.D., McNee R.K., Alley P.G., Woodfield D.G. (1985) Relation between cancer of the colon and blood transfusion, *Br. Med. J.* 290: 1826.

Graves T.A., Cioffi W.G., Mason A.D., McManus W.F., Pruitt B.A. (1989) Relationship of transfusion and infection in a burn population, *J. Trauma* 29: 948-954.

Jakobsen E.B., Eickhoff J.H., Andersen J., Lundvall L., Stenderup J.K. (1990) Perioperative blood transfusion and recurrence and death after resection cancer of the colon and rectum, *Scan. J. Gastroenterol.* 25: 435-442.

Jensen L.S., Andersen A.J., Christiansen P.M. et al. (1992) Postoperative infection and natural killer cell function following blood transfusion in patients undergoing elective colorectal surgery, *Br. J. Surg.* 79: 513-516.

Kaplan J., Sarnaik S., Gitlin J., Lusher J. (1984) Diminished helper/suppressor lymphocyte ratios and natural killer activity in recipients of repeated blood transfusions, *Blood* 64: 308-310.

Lawick van Pabst W.P., Langenhorst B., Mulder P., Marquet R.L., Jeekel J. (1988) Effect of perioperative blood loss and perioperative transfusions on colorectal cancer survival, *Eur. J. Cancer* 24: 741-747.

Liewald F., Wirshing R.P., Zulke C., Demmel N., Mempel W. (1990) Influence of blood transfusions on tumor recurrence and survival rate in colorectal carcinoma, *Eur. J. Cancer* 26: 327-335.

Mecklin J.P., Jarvinen J., Ovaska J.T. (1989) Blood transfusion and prognosis in colorectal carcinoma, *Scand. J. Gastroenterol.* 24: 33-39.

Mezrow C.K., Bergstein I., Tartter P.I. (1992) Post-operative infections following autologous and homologous blood transfusions, *Transfusion* 32: 27-30.

Miholic J., Hudec M., Domanig E. et al. (1985) Risk factors for severe bacterial infections after valve replacement and aortocoronary bypass operations: analysis of 246 cases by logistic regression, *Ann. Thorac. Surg.* 40: 224-228.

Murphy P., Heal J.M., Blumberg N. (1991) Infected or suspected infection after hip replacement surgery with autologous or homologous blood transfusions, *Transfusion* 31: 212-217.

Nagarkatti P.S., Joseph S., Singal D.P. (1983) Induction of antibodies by blood transfusions capable of inhibiting responses in MLC, *Transplantation* 36: 695-699.

Nathanson S.D., Tilley B.C., Schultz L., Smith R.F. (1985) Perioperative allogeneic blood transfusions. Survival in patients with resected carcinomas of the colon and rectum, *Arch. Surg.* 120: 734-738.

Opelz G., Sengar D.P.S., Mickey M.R., Terasaki P. (1973) Effect of blood transfusions on subsequent kidney transplants, *Transplant Proc.* 5: 253-259.

Ota D., Alvarez L., Lichtiger B., Giacco G., Guinee V. (1985) Perioperative blood transfusion in patients with colon carcinoma, *Transfusion* 25: 392-394.

Ottino G., De Paulis R., Pansini S. et al. (1987) Major sternal wound infection after open heart surgery: a multivariate analysis of risk factors in 2579 consecutive operative procedures, *Ann. Thorac. Surg.* 44: 173-179.

Parrott N.R. (1993) Blood transfusion: should we avoid it in our cancer patients?, *Current Practice in Surgery* 5: 127-131.

Parrott N.R., Lennard T.W.J., Taylor R.M.R., Proud G., Shenton B.K., Johnson I.D.A. (1986) Effect of perioperative blood transfusion on recurrence of colorectal cancer, *Br. J. Surg.* 73: 970-973.

Quintiliani L., Buzzonetti A., Digirolamo M. et al. (1991) Effects of blood transfusion on immune responsiveness and survival of cancer patients: a prospective study, *Transfusion* 31: 713-718.

Ross W.B. (1987) Blood transfusion and colorectal cancer, *J. Roy. Coll. Surg. Edin.* 32: 197-201.

Stephan R.N., Kisala J.N., Dean R.E., Geha A.S., Chaudry I.H. (1988) Effect of blood transfusion on autigen presentation function and on interleukin 2 generation, *Arch. Surg.* 123: 235-240.

Tartter P.I., Burrows L., Papatestas A., Lesnick G., Aufses A.H. (1985) Perioperative blood transfusion has prognostic significance for breast cancer, *Surgery* 97: 225-229.

Tartter P.I. (1988) Blood transfusion and infectious complications following colorectal cancer surgery, *Br. J. Surg.* 75: 789-792.

Tartter P.I., Driefuss R.M., Malon A.M., Keimann T.M., Aufses A.H. (1988) Relationship of postoperative septic complications and blood transfusions in patients with Crohns disease, *Am. J. Surg.* 155: 43-48.

Triulzi D.J., Vanek K., Ryan D.H., Blumberg N. (1992) A clinical and immunologic study of blood transfusion and postoperative bacterial infection in spinal surgery, *Transfusion* 32: 517-524.

Vamvakas E., Moore S.B. (1993) Perioperative blood transfusion and colorectal cancer recurrence: a qualitative statistical overview and meta-analysis, *Transfusion* 33: 754-765.

Vente J.P., Wiggers T., Weidema W.F., Jeekel J., Obertop H. (1989) Perioperative blood transfusion in colorectal cancer, *Eur. J. Surg. Oncol.* 15: 371-374.

Voogt P.J., Van de Velde C.J., Brand A. et al. (1987) Perioperative blood transfusion and cancer prognosis. Different effects of blood transfusion on prognosis of colon and breast cancer patients, *Cancer* 59: 836-843.

Waymack J.P., Balakrishnan K., McNeal N. et al. (1986) Effect of blood transfusions on macrophage-lymphocyte interaction in an animal model, *Ann. Surg.* 204: 681-685.

Waymack J.P., Callon L., Barcelli U., Trocki O., Alexander J.W. (1987) Effect of blood transfusions on immune function III. Alterations in macrophage arachidonic acid metabolism, *Arch. Surg.* 122: 56-60.

Weiden P.L., Bean M.A., Schultz P. (1987) Perioperative blood transfusion does not increase the risk of colorectal cancer recurrence, *Cancer* 60: 870-874.

Wobbes T., Joosens K.H., Kuypers H.H., Beerthuizen G.I., Theeuwes G.M. (1989) The effect of packed cells and whole blood transfusions on survival after curative resection for colorectal carcinoma, *Dis. Colon, Rectum* 32: 743-748.

The CMV Problem: The Role of Leucocyte Depletion in Minimising the Risk of CMV Transmission in Transfusion Medicine

11 | M. Böck and M.U. Heim

In assessing the role of leucocyte depletion in reducing the transmission of Cytomegalovirus as a result of transfusion, a review of recent published studies has been made and conclusions based on the findings of these studies will be presented in this paper.

The findings of workers in the mid-seventies using even low rates of leucocyte reduction, led subsequent researchers to examine the possibility of eliminating CMV transmission when higher rates of white cell reduction became possible using leucocyte removal filters.

It can be seen that CMV transmission can be avoided by the use of commercially available white cell depletion filters.

CMV Infection

Cytomegalovirus (CMV) is a human viral pathogen belonging to the family of Herpes viruses. It is a labile virus, which is readily inactivated by lipid solvents, acid, heat (37°C for one hour) and ultraviolet light. Primary infections in immunocompetent hosts are usually asymptomatic or subclinical and manifest as CMV seropositivity. By contrast, in immunocompromised patients CMV infection may cause serious morbidity including interstitial pneumonia, hepatitis, encephalitis, leucopenia and thrombocytopenia. Those considered at greatest risk are neonates and transplant patients. Lifelong infection characterised by latency of the virus with the possibility of reactivation generally follows the primary infection.

Epidemiologic studies have shown, that CMV infection is an ubiquitous phenomenon. The prevalence of antibodies in adults ranges from 40-100% depending on the socioeconomic conditions. Whereas in Europe, Australia and parts of South America a low prevalence could be demonstrated (e.g. Freiburg 42%, Melbourne 54%, Albany 45%), it is significantly higher in developing countries such as Africa or Southeast Asia (e.g. Entebbe 100%, Manila 100%) (Ho 1990).

Analysis of age related incidence of infection reveals two age brackets wherein increased infection occurs. The first is the perinatal period; 36-56% of infants are infected during the first year (Stagno et al. 1975). Sources of infections are virus transmission from passage through the birth canal, from CMV-containing milk by breast-feeding or banked milk and from other children in the newborn nursery, day care centres and within the family. The second is the period of sexual maturity since the uterine cervix and semen are important reservoirs of CMV and common sites of infection.

Iatrogenic viral transmission

The most important source of iatrogenic viral transmission is blood transfusion. It was first reported by Kaariainen et al. (1966), that blood transfusions implicate the risk of CMV transmission. In the early seventies Henle et al. (1970) suggested a coincidence between CMV infection and the number of transfused blood units. Prince et al. (1971) estimated an overall risk of 2.4 sero-conversions per 100 units transfused. In the interim many reports confirmed blood transfusions as an important source of disease transmission. In contrast to cellular blood products, however, transmission of CMV by fresh frozen plasma has not yet been proven (Bowden and Sayers 1990, Adler 1988).

Administration of CMV-seronegative blood products can prevent CMV transmission. This has been demonstrated in bone marrow transplant patients as well as in neonates (Miller et al. 1991, Mackinnon et al. 1988, Tegtmeier 1988, Benson et al. 1979, Bowden et al. 1987). The exclusive administration of CMV-seronegative blood products to all patients, however, would eliminate an unacceptable number of blood units and endanger the routine supply of red blood cells. Therefore, most centres reserve seronegative red blood cells for those patients having the greatest risk of serious CMV-infections such as transplant patients and premature infants.

Role of leucocytes (WBC) in CMV transmission

There is evidence suggesting that CMV is transmitted by viable leucocytes: Rates of infections in patients receiving unscreened WBC-transfusions are extraordinarily high. Blood components free of, or minimally contaminated with WBCs exhibit no, or clearly a reduced risk of transmitting CMV. Bowden and Sayers (1990) demonstrated that none of 21 seronegative marrow transplant recipients who underwent plasma exchange with unscreened plasma, showed evidence of infection either by culture or seroconversion. Neonates given washed red blood cells had lower rates of CMV infection than those receiving unwashed blood (Luban et al. 1987). Frozen deglycerolized red blood cells are characterised by a reduced risk of CMV transmission in dialysis patients (Tolkoff-Rubin et al. 1978).

Furthermore, Schrier et al. (1985) reported the detection of CMV-RNA in peripheral blood lymphocytes of seropositive individuals. Early CMV-antigens have been demonstrated in WBCs and in vitro replication of the virus was observed in peripheral blood T-cells (Rice et al. 1984, Einhorn and Ost 1984). From these data, it was proposed that removal of WBCs in transfused blood products would minimise the risk of CMV transmission.

Clinical Studies

The following table summarises the literature review and demonstrates the results of some clinical studies concerning the primary CMV infection in immunocompromised patients after WBC depleted and non-WBC depleted blood transfusions.

Transfusion associated infections

Author	Non-WBC depleted blood	WBC depleted blood
Lang D. et al. (1977)	4/6	2/8
Frank U. et al. (1987)	2/26	0/27
Verdonck L. et al. (1987)	-	0/29
Murphy S. et al. (1988)	2/9	0/11
De Graan H. et al. (1989)	10/86	0/59
Gilbert G. et al. (1989)	9/46	0/30
De Witte T. et al. (1990)	-	0/28
Eisenfeld L. et al. (1992)	-	0/48

Values give numbers of patients infected out of total patients.

In 1977 Lang et al. (Lang et al. 1977) reported data comparing patients having undergone cardiopulmonary bypass surgery receiving leucocyte depleted blood and whole blood. Leucocyte depletion was performed by differential centrifugation. The reduction rate averaged 42%. Despite this low white cell reduction a clear effect on CMV transmission could be demonstrated. In the control group four of six patients showed seroconversion. However, CMV transmission could be detected in only two of eight patients receiving leucocyte depleted red cells (this 25% infection rate probably results from the high amount of residual white cells in the transfused units).

Frank and Sugg (1987) demonstrated in 1987, that in none out of 27 surgical patients receiving leucocyte depleted blood (WBC reduction rate > 98%) could CMV transmission be demonstrated. In the control group however, two out of 26 patients were infected. The authors concluded that, although this difference was not statistically significant, it confirms the hypothesis of reduced CMV transmission after leucocyte depletion.

Verdonck et al. (1987) confirmed these results in patients undergoing bone marrow transplantation. In none out of 29 seronegative patients receiving filtered blood products was seroconversion observed. Similar results were obtained by the following researchers: Murphy et al. (1988) in acute leukaemia patients, De

Graan-Hentzen et al. (1989) in leukaemia and non-Hodgkin's lymphoma patients and De Witte et al. (1990) in bone marrow transplant patients.

In all these studies none of the patients receiving filtered blood products developed CMV seroconversion or other signs of infection. When newborn infants and neonatals with very low birth weight were included in the studies, the same results were obtained: no transmission of CMV was observed when leucocyte depleted blood products were administered (Gilbert et al. 1989, Eisenfeld et al. 1992). These results are in good agreement with observations of Smith et al., who could demonstrate by PCR technique, that filtration of red blood cells is successful in removing CMV-DNA from the samples (Smith et al. 1993).

Summary and conclusion

A large percentage of the population (50%-100%) carries CMV antibodies. In immunocompetent hosts, infection is usually asymptomatic or subclinical. In immuno-compromised patients however, serious morbidity may result from exposure to CMV infection. Transfusion of leucocyte containing blood products is an important source of iatrogenic viral transmission.

Such transfusion acquired CMV infection can be prevented by leucodepleting cellular blood products. Using the currently available high performance (4 log) filters capable of removing up to 99.99% of WBC, leucodepleted products of high quality can now be obtained. Such filtered products provide an alternative to CMV-negative blood for immunocompromised patients.

References

Adler S.P. (1988) Data that suggest that FFP does not transmit CMV (letter), *Transfusion* 28: 604.
Benson J.W., Bodden S.J., Tobin J. (1979) Cytomegalovirus and blood transfusion in neonates, *Arch. Dis. Child* 54: 538-541.
Bowden R., Sayers M. (1990) The risk of transmitting infection by fresh frozen plasma, *Transfusion* 30: 762-763.
Bowden R.A., Sayers M., Gleaves C.A. et al. (1987) Cytomegalovirus-seronegative blood components for the prevention of primary cytomegalovirus infection after marrow transplantation, *Transfusion* 27: 478-481.
De Graan-Hentzen Y.C.E., Gratama J.W., Mudde G.C. et al. (1989) Prevention of primary cytomegalovirus infection in patients with hematologic malignancies by intensive white cell depletion of blood products, *Transfusion* 29: 757-760.
De Witte T., Schattenberg A., Van Dijk B.A. et al. (1990) Prevention of primary cytomegalovirus infection after allogenic bone marrow transplantation by using leucocyte-poor random blood products from cytomegalovirus-unscreened blood-bank donors, *Transplant.* 50: 964-968.
Einhorn L., Ost A. (1984) Cytomegalovirus infection of human cells, *Jnl. Infect. Dis.* 149: 207-214.

Eisenfeld L., Silver H., McLaughlin J. et al. (1992) Prevention of transfusion-associated cyto-megalovirus infection in neonatal patients by the removal of white cells from blood, *Transfusion* 32 (3): 205-209.

Frank U., Sugg U. (1987) Gelingt mit leukozytenarmem Blut eine Reduktion der CMV-Infektion?, *Beitr. Infusionstherapie klin. Ernähr.* 18: 35-36.

Gilbert G.L., Hayes K., Hudson I. et al. (1989) Prevention of transfusion-acquired cytomegalo-virus infection in infants by blood filtration to remove leucocytes, *Lancet*, 1228-1231.

Henle W., Henle G., Scriba M. et al. (1970) Antibody responses to Epstein-Barr virus and cyto-megaloviruses after open-heart and other surgery, *New Engl. J. Med.* 282: 1068-1074.

Ho M. (1990) Epidemiology of Cytomegalovirus Infections, *Rev. Infect. Dis.* 12 (Suppl. 7): 701-710.

Kaariainen L., Klemola E., Paloheimo J. (1966) Rise of cytomegalovirus antibodies in an infec-tious-mononucleosis-like syndrome after transfusion. *Br. Med. J.* 2: 1270-1272.

Lang D.J., Ebert P.A., Rodgers B.M. et al. (1977) Reduction of postperfusion cytomegalovirus-infections following the use of leucocyte depleted blood, *Transfusion* 17: 391-395.

Luban N., Williams A., McDonald M. et al. (1987) Low incidence of acquired cytomegalovirus infection in neonates transfused with washed red blood cells, *AJDC* 141: 416-419.

Mackinnon S., Burnett A.K., Crawford R.J. et al. (1988) Seronegative blood products prevent primary cytomegalovirus infection after bone marrow transplantation, *J. Clin. Pathol.* 41: 948-950.

Miller W.J., McCullough J., Balfour H.H. et al. (1991) Prevention of cytomegalovirus infection following bone marrow transplantation: a randomised trial of blood product screening, *Bone Marrow Transplant.* 7: 227-234.

Murphy M.F., Grint P.C.S.A., Hardiman A.E. et al. (1988) Use of leucocyte-poor blood compo-nents to prevent primary cytomegalovirus (CMV) infection in patients with acute leukaemia, *Br. J. Haematol.* 70: 253-254.

Prince A.M., Szmuness W., Millian S.J. et al. (1971) A serologic study of cytomegalovirus infec-tions associated with blood transfusions, *N. Engl. J. Med.* 284: 1125-1131.

Rice G.P.A., Schrier R.D., Oldstone M.B.A. (1984) Cytomegalovirus infects human lymphocytes and monocytes: virus expression is restricted to immediate-early gene prod-ucts, *Proc. Natl. Acad. Sci.* 81: 6134-6138.

Schrier R.D., Nelson J.A., Oldstone M.B.A. (1985) Detection of human cytomegalovirus in peripheral blood lymphocytes in a natural infection, *Science* 230: 1048-1051.

Smith K.L., Cobain T., Dunstan R.A. (1993) Removal of cytomegalo-virus DNA from donor blood by filtration, *Br. J. Haematol.* 83: 640-642.

Stagno S., Reynolds D.W., Tsiantos A. et al. (1975) Comparative serial virologic and serologic studies of symptomatic and subclinical congenitally and natally acquired cytomegalovirus infections, *J. Infect. Dis.* 132: 568-577.

Tegtmeier G.E. (1988) The use of cytomegalovirus-screened blood in neonates, *Transfusion* 28: 201-203.

Tolkoff-Rubin N.E., Rubin R.H., Keller E.E. et al. (1978) Cytomegalovirus infection in dialysis patients and personnel, *Ann. Intern. Med.* 89: 625-628.

Verdonck L.F., De Graan-Hentzen Y.C.E., Dekker A.W. et al. (1987) Cytomegalovirus seronegative platelets and leucocyte-poor red blood cells from random donors can prevent primary cytomegalovirus infection after bone marrow transplantation, *Bone Marrow Trans-plant.* 2: 73-78.

Development of Anti-HLA Antibodies in Multiply Transfused Preterm Infants

12 | R.P.A. Rivers

Much attention has been given in recent years to the assessment and improvement of tissue oxygen delivery in the very low birthweight, preterm infant by optimising the red cell mass (Jones et al. 1990). One identified cause of a reduction in the 'ideal' red cell mass is the practice of early cord clamping at delivery in order to facilitate resuscitation of the baby and to reduce body cooling. The consequence of the prevention of this potential transfusion of placental blood along with the repeated blood losses via venesection for investigational purposes has been the finding of a low red cell mass in many such infants together with a frequent need for donor blood transfusion (Kinmond et al. 1993). One measure that has been researched in regard to reducing the number of donor transfusions required has been the use of erythropoietin given along with iron and, on occasion, protein supplementation. However until methods for facilitating placental transfusion at delivery of these babies are further explored, many are going to require the infusion of red cells, at least in the early weeks of life.

HLA antigens, otherwise known as the major histocompatibility complex antigens, are the most important in determining the compatibility of tissue grafts. HLA-A, HLA-B and HLA-C antigens are present on platelets and all nucleated cells except placental trophoblasts and spermatozoa. It is these antigens, present on T lymphocytes, that are detectable in lymphocytoxicity assays. In addition to the above cell types, HLA antigens including HLA B7, B17, A2 and B8 have been described as being expressed on red blood cells.

Complications arising from transfusions in these VLBW infants who make up the majority of the neonatal transfusion needs, may differ from those arising in babies receiving relatively large donor volumes as during in utero or in exchange transfusion procedures. Of particular relevance in the pathogenesis of possible complications is the capacity of the immune system to respond to foreign antigens; these are processed and linked to HLA class II antigens by donor presenting cells, for recognition by the recipient's helper (CD4) lymphocytes. Although the helper - suppressor ratio is found to be increased in term and preterm infants compared with adults (Ballow et al. 1987), the strong suppressor activity of cord-derived T-lymphocytes contrasts with their mainly CD4 (helper) phenotype. It has been suggested that the CD4 neonatal cells are deficient in their ability to provide help for antibody production having this dominant suppressor immunoregulatory activity and that it is only when they undergo maturational changes that they become capable of helper function (Clement et al. 1990). The capacity to respond is considered to be more related to the duration of extra-uterine life than to gestational age at birth (Quie 1990). Sensitization to maternal leucocytes has been purported to occur with the production of alloantibodies to HLA antigens (Schroeder 1974) although alloimmunization to red blood cell antigens have only rarely been described. Their occurrence has been recently reviewed by Strauss (1993).

The principal known consequences of transfusing white blood cells include alloimmunization to cell antigens, febrile transfusion reactions, transmission of donor infection by white blood cell associated organisms, graft-versus host disease, prothrombotic tissue factor expression on donor monocytes, immune modulation and reduced pulmonary perfusion due to the deposition of activated granulocytes in the lung.

In the study by Bedford Russell et al. (1993), one objective was to establish whether multiply transfused preterm infants might be capable of antibody production to transfused foreign HLA antigens. Previous studies had used different methods for antibody detection and in one described instance where HLA - A1 antibody positivity was documented, it was suggested that the infant had been immunised to maternal HLA-A1 in utero since the donor blood which had been used in transfusion had been negative for this antigen (Rawls et al. 1984). Two other studies have indicated that intrauterine immunisation to maternal white cells can occur. In one the cord antibodies could be adsorbed by maternal but not paternal lymphocytes (Chardonnens et al. 1980) and in the other antibodies were present in 5 of 62 cord specimens which reacted with lymphocyte or granulocyte antigens (Mathur et al. 1981). Whilst maternal HLA antibodies developing in a pregnancy in response to paternal haplotypes would not be expected to cross the placenta, such antibodies when having their origins in a previous pregnancy or in response to a previous blood transfusion can be found in cord sera. In the study (Bedford Russell et al. 1993) of 53 babies admitted to a neonatal unit at less than 37 weeks gestation, results were available on 42 who subsequently received at least 2 transfusions. In 11 of the mother-infant pairs, anti-HLA antibodies (a-HLA) were detected in the mother but not in the paired baby cord sample; in 3 babies (2 of whom were twins) a-HLA were found in cord sera but sera were unavailable from the respective mothers; in 2 of these, the antibodies disappeared by one month of age. In only one infant was an a-HLA shown to be present which corresponded to an antibody in the mother. This antibody was no longer detectable in the infant one month later.

Returning to the question as to whether postnatal transfusions in a group of preterm babies could induce a-HLA, two groups of infants were studied. 19 were of gestational age range 24-35 weeks (mean 29) and these received their transfusions through an in-line white cell depleting filter. A further 23 infants, who received their transfusions without any such filter, were of a gestational range 24 - 36 weeks (mean 29). The 'in-line' leucocyte removal microfilter used to render the donor blood leucocyte and platelet reduced was composed of non-woven polyester fibres adapted from the standard Sepacell (Asahi Medical Company Japan) and designed for use with up to 50 ml donor blood. Red cell recovery was between 95.7-100% (n = 10) and the absolute WBC was between 0.1-0.3x10^9/L (n = 10). The filter group received rather more transfusions: 8 (range 2-35) compared with 4 (range 2-22) in the no filter group. Whilst no babies developed antibodies in the filter group, 7 of the 23 in the no filter group developed one or more a-HLA which, in the one case where passive maternal antibody had been found in cord serum, was of a different HLA specificity. In most instances the antibodies had disappeared within one or more months after their initial detection although in one instance, multi-specific antibodies were detected sequentially being still present at 4 months. Although the significance of these findings has been questioned (Strauss 1993) in view of the transient nature of their presence and the lack of evident clinical effects, in no instances were the babies receiving repeated transfusions of the same donor blood. Recently, with improved storage capability utilising multipacs and new media which may enable red cells to be given after some 4 or more weeks of storage, a given baby may be electively protected from multiple donor exposure, receiving repeated exposures to a single donor by intent. In the study situation, it would have been unlikely for an infant to be exposed multiply to a previously encountered HLA thereby reducing the opportunity for both antibody persistence or transfusion reaction. With this recently advocated change in transfusion protocol, the opportunity for repeated stimulation by the same donor white blood cell HLA containing blood is inevitable. The question then arises as to whether the presence of specific antibodies would be clinically relevant.

Transfusion reactions
It is likely to be difficult to recognise transfusion reactions in preterm infants where apnoea, temperature instability, deterioration in pulmonary function, peripheral mottling and altered behaviour, although possibly indicative of such an occurrence, are non-specific. Indeed, such changes in clinical status in very preterm infants are common and their true causation, even if linked with a transfusion, may remain unappreciated. Prospective studies are required to answer this question. Haemolytic transfusion reactions may also occur in the presence of a-HLA when the HLA is expressed on red cells. Shortened red cell survival has been reported in a group of adults transfused with HLA incompatible blood (Panzer et al. 1987). In particular HLA-B7 incompatibility was studied and it is of interest that in two of the infants reported in the Bedford Russell study, HLA B7 was the antibody identified. It is not infrequent to observe a failure of red cell transfusion to achieve a sustained rise in haemoglobin level in preterm infants; whether this is ever a consequence of the shortened survival of donor cells in the presence of a-HLA remains to be established.

Graft versus host disease
GVHD is a complication following the infusion of histo-incompatible lymphoid cells; in view of the alleged impaired cellular immunity of the preterm and newborn infant, it might be anticipated that such a disease would be common following neonatal transfusions. When GVHD occurs in the immunocompetent individ-

ual, it is believed to arise as a consequence of the blood being from a donor homozygous for one of the recipients HLA haplotypes. This results in the failure of recognition of foreign major histocompatibility - complex antigens with a failure to develop an immune response. This is particularly likely in transfusions between first degree relatives, estimated at 1 in 475 of such transfusions (Ohto et al. 1992). However, the rarity of GVHD occurrence in neonatal transfusions, although in part resulting from the practice of gamma irradiation of cellular blood products in certain countries, may be more commonly the result of a gradual diminution in the donor-anti-host response due to suppression of this response by host-derived T cells (Mast et al. 1994). Identified risk factors for the development of GVHD include intrauterine and exchange transfusions where the volume of donor white blood cells is relatively large, severe immunodeficiency and transfusions from first degree relatives. The only case cited by Strauss (1993) which occurred outside the above risk groups was that of an extremely premature infant (Sanders et al. 1990). The potential dangers of gamma irradiation include DNA injury and the possibility of leukaemic transformation. White blood cell reduction by filter for at risk groups to a load level of $< 10^5$ per kilo might seem more rational since this number of white cells has not been shown to be associated with the development of GVHD. For large volumes, the removal of microaggregates at the same time could be regarded as beneficial.

In summary it would seem justifiable to reduce white blood cells and aggregates in blood being used for exchange transfusions in the neonatal period or where the risks of developing GVHD have been identified; this should include transfusions from first degree relatives. The routine reduction of white blood cells in small volume transfusions to reduce the risk of CMV transmission in unidentified infectious donors and of other infectious agents which might be present remains controversial. In balancing the high cost of intensive care given to these high risk babies against the potential low cost of an in-line filter which could be used for the relatively few small-volume top-up transfusions which such a baby is likely to require, it would appear irrational to expose these infants to the risk of possible CMV or other organism transmission particularly when the associated high mortality and morbidity from CMV in this group of patients is so well established. The consequences of a-HLA production in this group of infants in causing transfusion reactions remains to be further investigated.

References

Ballow M., Cates K.L., Rowe J.C., Goatz C., Pantschenko A.G. (1987) Peripheral blood T-cell subpopulations in the very low birth weight (less than 1,500 g) infant, *Amer. J. Hemat.* 24: 85-92.

Bedford Russell A.R., Rivers R.P.A., Davey, N. (1993) The development of anti-HLA antibodies in multiply transfused preterm infants, *Arch. Dis. Child.* 68: 49-51.

Chardonnens, X., Jeannet, M. (1980) Immunobiology of pregnancy: evidence for fetal immune response against the mother, *Tissue Antigens* 15: 401-406.

Clement L.T., Vink P.E., Bradley, G.E. (1990) Novel immunoregulatory functions of phenotypically distinct subpopulations of CD4+ cells in the human neonate, *J. Immunol.* 145: 102-108.

Jones J.G., Holland B.M., Hudson I.R.B., Wardrop C.A.J. (1990) Total circulating red cells versus haematocrit as the primary descriptor of oxygen transport by the blood, *Br. J. Haematol.* 76: 288-294.

Kinmond S., Aitchison T.C., Holland B.M., Jones J.C., Turner T.L., Wardrop C.A.J. (1993) Umbilical cord clamping and preterm infants: a randomised trial, *Brit. Med. J.* 306: 172-175.

Mast B.J. van der, Hornstra N., Ruigrok M.B., Claas F.H.J., Rood J.J van, Lagaaij E.L. (1994) Transfusion-associated graft-versus-host disease in immunocompetent patients: a self-protective mechanism, *Lancet* 343: 753-757.

Mathur S., Keane M., Williamson H.O., Bulusu L.K., Little F.M., Tucker M.L., Rust P.F., Fudenberg H.H. (1981) Antibodies to sperm, ovary, B and T lymphocytes, and granulocytes in the umbilical circulation and in newborn infants, *Clin. Immunol. Immunopathol.* 20: 116-122.

Ohto H., Yasuda H., Noguchi M. (1992) Risk of transfusion-associated graft-versus-host disease as a result of directed donations from relatives, *Transfusion* 32: 691-693.

Panzer S., Mayr W.R., Graninger W., Puchler K., Hocker P., Lechner K. (1987) Haemolytic transfusion reactions due to HLA antibodies, *Lancet* i: 474-478.

Quie P.G. (1990) Antimicrobial defenses in the neonate, *Sem. in Perinatol.* 14 (4) (Suppl. 1): 2-9.

Rawls W.E., Wong C.L., Blajchman M., Venturelli J., Watts J., Chernesky M., Saigal S. (1984) Neonatal cytomegalovirus infections: the relative role of neonatal bloodtransfusion and maternal exposure, *Clin. Invest. Med.* 7: 13-19.

Sanders M.R., Graeber J.E. (1990) Post transfusion graft-versus-host disease in infancy, *J. Pediatr.* 117: 159-163.

Schroeder J. (1974) Passage of leukocytes from mother to fetus, *Scand. J. Immunol.* 3: 369-373.

Strauss R.G. (1993) Selection of white cell-reduced blood components for transfusions during early infancy, *Transfusion* 33: 352-357.

Failure of Leucocyte Filtration - Does it occur?

13 G. Berlin and E. Ledent

Introduction

Leucocyte filtration is commonly used to avoid transfusion complications caused by leucocyte contamination of the blood products, e.g. non-hemolytic febrile transfusion reactions, transmission of intracellular viruses and bacteria, and allo-immunization to HLA-antigens. The number of cells needed to induce HLA-immunization is unknown but several reports indicate that transfusing blood products containing $<10^6$ leucocytes/unit prevents immunization (Saarinen et al. 1990, Oksanen et al. 1991). European guidelines state that a filtered erythrocyte concentrate should contain $<5 \times 10^6$ leococytes. It should be pointed out that even a single transfusion with a higher number of contaminating leucocytes might cause HLA-immunization. Consequently, a strict quality control should be performed to ensure an efficient leucocyte filtration. This might be difficult to do in daily work as leucocyte filtration often is performed bed-side at the ward, with the filter inserted in the transfusion administration line.

After having used bed-side leucocyte filtration of all blood products transfused to patients with hematogical malignancies for more than a year we did not notice any obvious reduction in the frequency of the platelet refractory state at our hospital. To find a reason for this we decided to improve our quality control of bed-side filtration. This was done by counting the number of leucocytes after transfusion of erythrocyte concentrates in a segment of the transfusion tubing line situated directly under the filter. We then found a surprisingly high number of cells (median 386×10^6/l, range: $<10^5$-5×10^9, n=28), a finding that could not be reproduced when filtering under laboratory conditions.

The main difference between the two filtration methods is the flow rate; at the bed-side the filtration is completed in 1-2 h whereas the filtration in the laboratory is performed at fast flow (by gravity, approximately 10 min). We therefore investigated the efficiency of leucocyte filtration under bed-side and laboratory conditions, and the influence of the composition of the blood product on the filtration result.

Materials and methods

450 ml blood from healthy donors was collected in CPD and left at room temperature for 2-12 h. After centrifugation at 2500 g for 12 min the blood was divided into plasma, buffy coat and erythrocytes suspended in 100 ml SAGMAN

solution (RBC). The RBCs were stored at +4°C over-night and kept at room temperature for approximately 10 min prior to filtration.

The number of leucocytes was counted in a Bürker chamber (prefiltration sample) and in a Nageotte chamber (postfiltration sample, bed-side filters) or by flow cytometry (Epics Profile I; postfiltration sample, blood bank filters). A differential count of polymorphonuclear (PMN) and mononuclear cells was performed.

Comparison of filtration at fast and slow flow using bed-side filters.
The filters used in the study were: RC50 and RC100 (PALL Corp.), Sepacell R200 and R500 (Asahi Medical Co.) and Erypur Optima b (Organon Teknika). One unit of RBC was filtered through each filter. The filtration was performed either at fast flow (by gravity, approx. 10 min) or at slow flow (approx. 2 h). Rinsing of the filter with saline was done only when using Erypur Optima b as recommended by the manufacturer in order to reduce the RBC volume loss.

Study of blood bank filters at fast flow.
RBCs were filtered at fast flow (by gravity; approx. 10 min) through the following filters: BPF4 (PALL Corp.), RS200 (Asahi Medical Co.) and BioR01 plus (Biofil).

Influence of plasma on leucocyte filtration efficiency.
Two units of ABO-compatible whole blood were pooled, mixed and split into two equal parts; a test unit and a control unit. The control RBC was suspended in 100 ml of SAGMAN solution whereas 5 or 10 ml of SAGMAN was substituted with an equal amount of autologous plasma in the test unit. The filtration was performed through a RC50 filter (PALL Corp.) at a slow flow rate (2 h).

Results

Prior to filtration our RBCs contained 600×10^6 leucocytes (median, range: 120-1400×10^6) with 95% PMNs.

Comparison of filtration at fast and slow flow using bed-side filters.
As shown in Table 1 the RBCs filtered at slow flow had a significantly higher leucocyte contamination than RBCs filtered at fast flow. The majority (77%) of units contained $>5 \times 10^6$ leucocytes after filtration at slow flow compared to 23% at fast flow (all filters taken together). The increased postfiltration leucocyte number at slow flow was mainly caused by a high PMN number. There was also a significantly higher number of mononuclear cells/unit after filtration at slow flow compared to fast flow when using RC50 and R200.

Study of blood bank filters at fast flow.
The median postfiltration number of leucocytes was low for all tested filters and very few units contained $>5 \times 10^6$ leucocytes (Table 1). The percentage of units

with a leucocyte contamination below the detection limit of our flow cytometry method (0.1×10^6/l) was 46% for BPF4, 9% for RS200 and 44% for BioR01 plus.

Table 1 *Filtration of one-day old, buffy coat-reduced RBC units at fast or slow flow rate (post-filtration values). No 1-5 bed-side filters, no 6-8 blood bank filters*

Filter	Flow rate	Leucocytes $\times 10^6$/unit	Units with $> 5 \times 10^6$	PMN %
1. RC50	fast	2.4* (0.2-12.5)**	6/27	13
	slow	24.5 (0.9-192)	24/27	75
2. R200	fast	1.8 (0.8-8.2)	2/10	39
	slow	36.1 (10.5-121)	10/10	88
3. Erypur Optima b	fast	2.7 (0.3-13.7)	3/10	41
	slow	8.6 (1.7-14.6)	8/10	57
4. RC100	slow	5.0 (0.8-384)	5/10	n.d.
5. R500	slow	5.9 (0.8-25.4)	5/10	n.d.
6. BPF4	fast	0.02 (<0.02-2.99)	0/1300	n.d.
7. RS200	fast	0.17 (<0.02-7.12)	2/94	n.d.
8. BioR01 plus	fast	0.02 (<0.02-1.7)	0/54	n.d.

* Median
** range
PMN = polymorphonuclear cells
n.d. = not done

Influence of plasma on leucocyte filtration efficiency
The plasma volume of our control RBCs was calculated to 5.8 ± 2.9 ml (mean $\pm$ SD). There was no difference in pre-filtration number of leucocytes and platelets or the percentage of PMNs of the test and control units. When 5 or 10 ml of SAGMAN was substituted with an equal volume of autologous plasma (test units) we found a significant decrease in the post-filtration number of leucocytes (PMN and mononuclear cells) compared to the control units (Table 2).

Table 2 *The effect of substituting 5 or 10 ml of SAGMAN solution with an equal volume of autologous plasma (post-filtration values, RC50 filter at slow flow)*

Unit	5 ml plasma (n = 8)		10 ml plasma (n = 10)	
	Test unit	Control unit	Test unit	Control unit
Leucocytes x10^6/unit	6.85±6.75*	36.5±18.9	1.9±1.5	30.0±28.9
	p = 0.002		p = 0.013	
PMNs (%)	68.0±13	89.6±5.0	30.6±20	80.7±9.0
	p = 0.002		p < 0.001	

* mean±SD.

Discussion

In modern transfusion medicine we aim at transfusing blood products which are as 'pure' as possible. Leucocyte-reduced blood components can be achieved by filtration which for practical reasons often is performed bed-side during the transfusion. In this situation a slow flow rate is used compared to the fast gravity flow used when filtration is done at the blood bank. It has previously been reported that a filtration time of 2 h will not reduce the filtration efficiency compared to fast flow (Pikul et al. 1989). Testing several bed-side filters we found, however, a significantly higher number of leucocytes in RBCs filtered during 2 h compared to a short filtration time (10 min). Filtration through blood bank filters under standardized conditions at a fast flow rate resulted in a very good leucocyte depletion.

A high number of residual mononuclear cells (lymphocytes, monocytes and dendritic cells) might induce HLA-immunization while a high number of PMNs might cause viral or bacterial transmission. The mechanism of leucocyte depletion by filtration probably varies for different cell types. PMNs are thought to be removed mainly by adherence to the filter fibres while mononuclear cells are said to be removed by mechanical sieving (Steneker et al. 1991, Steneker et al. 1992). We found mainly a high number of PMNs after filtration at a slow flow rate but the number of mononuclear cells was also increased for some of the filters (RC50 and R200) suggesting that other mechanisms might be involved.

The composition of the RBC might be of importance for the filtration result. It has been claimed that platelets play a vital role in the filtration process mainly by removing PMNs through increased adherence and by microaggregate formation leading to cell trapping (Steneker et al. 1993). We used hard-packed, buffy coat-reduced RBCs with a low number of platelets (approx. 2x10^9/unit) and a low amount of plasma. When we altered the composition of the RBC by substituting 5 or 10 ml of the SAGMAN solution with an equal volume of autologous plasma we got a marked improvement in filtration efficiency. The residual number of PMNs as well as mononuclear cells decreased significantly in a volume-dependent manner compared to the control units. The mechanism by which the addition of a small amount of plasma improves the filtration efficiency is unknown. Only part of the plasma improvement was achieved by albumin (data not shown) suggesting something more than a general protein effect. The number of platelets was equal in the control RBCs and the test units.

Failure of leucocyte filtration - does it occur? Yes, it does occur! As shown in this study the efficiency of leucocyte filtration is influenced by factors such as flow rate and even minor differences in the composition of the blood product. It is thus important to perform quality control on a regular basis to assure that the filter has a good performance under all premises with the type of blood product to be used. This is more easily done at the blood bank compared to the bed-side situation.

References

Oksanen K., Kekomäki R., Ruutu T., Koskimies S., Myllylä G. (1991) Prevention of alloimmunization in patients with acute leukemia by use of white cell-depleted blod components - a randomized trial, *Transfusion* 31: 588-594.

Pikul F.J., Farrar P.R., Boris M.B., Estok L., Marlo D., Wildgen M., Chaplin H. (1989) Effectiveness of two synthetic fiber filters for removing white cells from AS-1 red cells, *Transfusion* 29: 590-595.

Saarinen U.M., Kekomäki R., Siimes M.A., Myllylä G. (1990) Effective prophylaxis against refractoriness in multitransfused patients by use of leukocyte-free blood components, *Blood* 75: 512-517.

Steneker I., Biewenga J. (1991) Histological and immunohistochemical studies on the preparation of white cell-poor red cell concentrates: the filtration process using three different polyester filters, *Transfusion* 31: 40-46.

Steneker I., Van Luyn M.J.A., Van Wachem P.B., Biewenga J. (1992) Electronmicroscopic examination of white cell reduction by four white cell-reduction filters, *Transfusion* 32: 450-457.

Steneker I., Prins H.K., Florie M., Loos J.A., Biewenga J. (1993) Mechanisms of leukocyte depletion of red cell concentrates by filtration. The effect of the cellular composition of the red cell concentrate, *Transfusion* 33: 42-50.

The Future of Leucocyte Depletion: In-line Filtration

14 | G. Matthes

The current situation for white cell depletion of red cell concentrates

The emergence of Transfusion Medicine as an independant branch of medicine has come in parallel with the development of blood component therapy. The principle of such specific haemotherapy is that only those blood components required are administered to the patient. With traditional blood bag technology one cannot avoid exposing the recipient of red cell concentrates (RCC) to donor leucocytes. Therefore different White Blood Cell (WBC) depletion methods have been developed and used. Filtration has been shown to be the most effective of these methods. The goal of WBC depletion of blood units is to reduce the donor white cells normally found in RCCs (about 10^9 per unit) to a level where undesirable effects of WBCs (and platelets) can be minimised or excluded (Klapper and Goldfinger 1992, Klein 1992).

Today, leucocyte filtration with modern filter materials allows a log 4 reduction of donor leucocytes. Bed-side filtration, as well as filtration in the bloodbank before transfusion, are current practice. The most recent development is an in-line filtration set (a blood bag system with integrated filter) wherein the blood components are separated as usual and subsequently filtered without the need for opening the system. This results in a series of advantages such as standardised blood component quality, no danger of contamination during subsequent filtration, no microaggregate formation, filtered units always being available, etc.. However, new questions are arising from this. For instance, when is the best time for filtration (immediately after donation or at a later time), should whole blood or separated red cells be filtered, what is the effect of the filtration on the quality of the red blood cells during storage.

Influence of in-line filtration on the storage ability of red cells

Until now no negative effects of filtration on the storage ability of red cells have been described. It was assumed moreover that, after filtration with the related reduction in potential toxic influence from leucocyte and platelet fragments, it should be possible to improve the preservation of red cells during the course of storage. To judge the viability and function of red cells usually only well-known parameters such as ATP, 2,3-DPG, free haemoglobin etc. have been employed (Hau 1993).

Our experiences* with the in-line blood bag system SEPACELL INTEGRA® (Diamed Transfusionstechnik GmbH Germany) confirm the assumption that filtration prior to storage can improve the in vitro function of red cells. The SEPACELL INTEGRA® blood bag systems evaluated were configured with four or five bags together with an integrated log 4 filter (Asahi Medical Co. Ltd., Japan) which was specifically designed for this purpose. Rapid and efficient white cell reduction was possible (residual WBC content $< 10^6$ per unit; average red cell loss $< 10\%$) (Müller et al. 1993).

Haemolysis parameters

In our examination of the in-line filtered red blood cells (SAG-M) over a storage period of 42 days at 4°C, no difference was observed compared to non-filtered RCCs produced under the current system (also resuspended in SAG-M). In addition to the haemolytic parameters (Hb, Hct, MCV, MCHC) we examined the free haemoglobin and potassium ion concentration in the supernatant. The level of haemolysis at the end of the storage time was less than 0.9%.

Metabolic parameters

Analysis of metabolic parameters (ATP, 2,3-DPG, Glucose consumption, Lactate accumulation, extra-cellular pH) of the stored red cells, revealed that the in-line filtered RCCs exhibited the same performance as non-filtered blood (Figure 1). In filtered red cells, the 2,3-DPG level measured during the first storage week was maintained for slightly longer than in non-filtered cells. One can assume this finding suggests a better oxygen transport function of the filtered cells. After 42 days the limit of acceptable storage time has been reached.

Parameters of oxygen transport function

Of specific interest for the efficacy of the transfusion, is the oxygen transport capability of the red cells. As an effective in vitro parameter of oxygen transport, the partial oxygen pressure of the haemoglobin (p50) was used, which reflects the oxygen dissociation curve. To assess the quality of the stored red cells we have, for the first time evaluated in in-line filtered RCCs, their real purpose: their ability to transport oxygen, and have found an interesting phenomenon (Matthes et al. 1993a).

---

* Results from the GEMUSEF STUDY (Berlin, Essen, Köln). This is a German, prospective, controlled, multi-centre study of storage and clinical use of red cell concentrates which have been obtained and processed using the Asahi Medical SEPACELL INTEGRA® system.

Figure 1 *Changes in intra-cellular ATP and 2,3-DPG as well as in Glucose and Lactate concentration in the supernatant during the 42 day storage of RBCs (SAG-M) after in-line filtration with the SEPACELL INTEGRA® system*

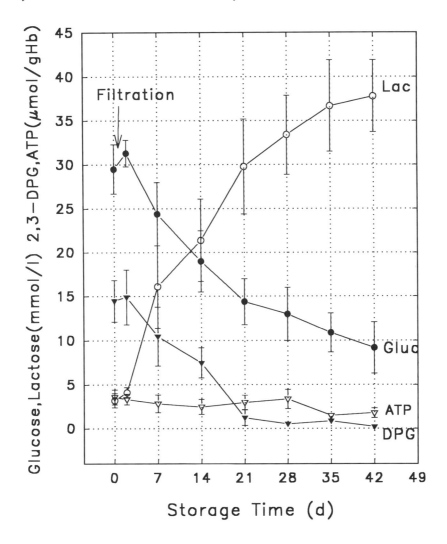

In non-filtered red cells the 2,3-DPG content declines over storage time, to less than 10% of the initial value, and as expected p50 declines, from 26-27 mm Hg to 15 mm Hg. For in-line filtered red cells such a correlation was not observed. With increasing storage time, p50 either remained stable or increased up to values of 30-35 mm Hg (Figure 2). Analysis of the haemoglobin derivatives oxyhaemoglobin and de-oxyhaemoglobin, confirmed this observation for in-line filtered blood, with the percentage of oxyhaemoglobin rising from 50-60% to in excess of 90% (Figure 3).

Figure 2 *Comparison between the kinetics of intracellular 2,3-DPG and p50 of in-line filtered RBCs (SAG-M) using the SEPACELL INTEGRA® system, and non-filtered RBCs (SAG-M) during 42 day storage*

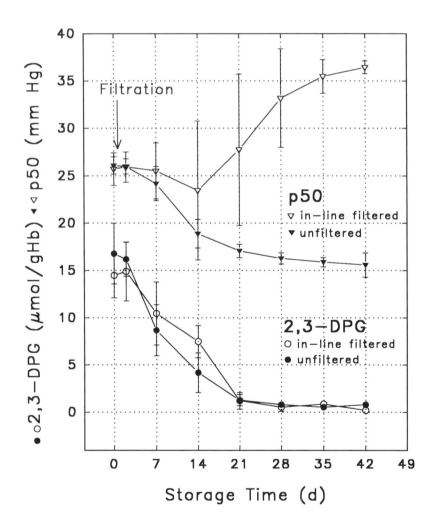

The reasons for the obtained oxygen transport capability of the stored red cells after in-line filtration are not fully understood. The following may contribute:

1. Cell Retention: During filtration of red cell concentrates older, rigid red cells are retained in the filter, therefore there is a relative increase in the content of younger cells.

2. Changes in Permeability: some of the proteins in the surrounding protein layer of the red cells may be bound to the filter materials changing the glyco-

calyx and resulting in a greater permeability to gases, electrolytes and other required substances which may influence the oxygen-binding capability of the haemoglobin.

3. White Blood Cell Elimination: because of WBC depletion there are no toxic effects from biologically active cell components released from degenerating leucocytes and platelets. However, in contrast to points 1 and 2, such WBC elimination is less likely to cause this p50-phenomenon because this same effect cannot be shown after repeated washing (log 3 reduction) of red blood cell concentrates.

Figure 3 *Changes of the haemoglobin derivatives (Oxy-Hb, Deoxy-Hb) during 42 day storage with in-line filtered RBCs (SAG-M) using the SEPACELL INTEGRA® system, compared to non-filtered RBCs (SAG-M)*

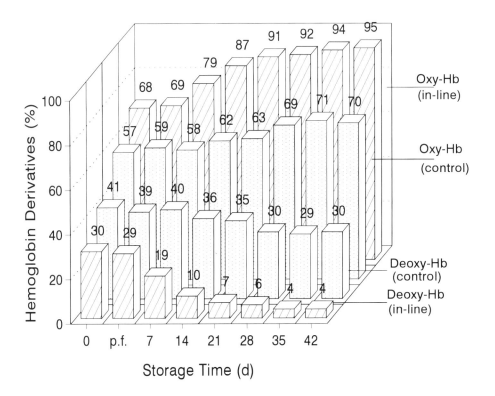

With continued scientific work on white cell depletion by filtration greater attention should be given not only to the mechanism of white cell depletion but also to the above mentioned phenomenon.

The effects of transfusing in-line filtered red cell concentrates

Assuming that the obtained in vitro oxygen transport function of the stored red cells persists in vivo, we analysed the performance of in-line filtered RCCs in patients, after transfusion. The RCCs (SAG-M) for transfusion, were prepared using the in-line technique, filtered within 6 hours after donation and then stored for up to 11 days. The control group was routine RCCs having been stored for a period of 11 days, and leucocyte depleted in the blood bank one day prior to transfusion. The RCCs were all resuspended in SAG-M.

Figure 4 shows the capillary p50 response in a total of 18 chronic anaemia patients, measured 20 minutes after the end of transfusion of two in-line filtered RCCs. This shows a similar response to the results obtained in previous studies of the in vivo regeneration of 2,3-DPG after transfusion of non-filtered red cell concentrates, resuspended in SAG-M and stored for 14 days (Matthes et al. 1993b).

Figure 4 *Differences in the capillary p50 values of patients (measured pre-transfusion and 20 minutes after the end of the transfusion of two in-line filtered RBCs (SAG-M)), plotted against the time lag between filtration and transfusion*

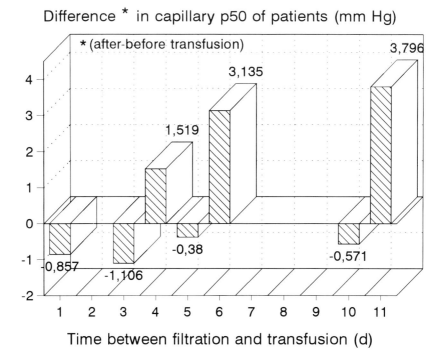

In the control group, the capillary p50 decreases and requires up to 24 hours to reach the original, pre-transfusion level. In contrast to this decrease, in-line filtered RCCs having been stored for a minimum of 4 days at 4°C, cause the p50 to increase in the patient. After transfusion of in-line filtered RCCs stored for 11 days, the capillary p50 measured in the patients' blood, increased by approximately 4 mm Hg.

This reveals a further and possibly more important advantage of in-line filtration: In addition to preventing the side effects which otherwise result from red cell transfusions contaminated with white cells, leucocyte depletion of blood units prior to storage can improve the efficacy of the transfusion.

New perspectives regarding the use of in-line filtered RCCs will emerge as even red cells stored for a longer period are capable of performing their oxygen transport function immediately after transfusion. Further clinical studies related to the efficacy of transfusion of in-line filtered blood will reveal if limitations related to storage time of red cell concentrates for specific indications (e.g. massive transfusions) or for patients with limited coronary, or cerebral limited coronary or cerebral compensation ablity, compensation ability can be removed. Additionally the question arises if due to these observed effects, the volume to be transfused can be reduced thus contributing to the saving of homologous blood donations.

Future possibilities of depletion/filtration

Depletion of leucocytes prior to the commencement of hypothermic storage is also leading to an exceptionally interesting possibility for improving the preservation of red cells. This arises from a modification or combination of different filter materials, by which one can not only achieve an in-line leucocyte depletion but also, for example a depletion of chloride ion in the red cell concentrates (Matthes et al. 1993c). Utilising this, the concept of long term storage with chloride free preservation solutions, as proposed by Meryman (Meryman et al. 1991), could be implemented without the need for storage in a large volume of preservation solution or for repeated washing.

Figure 5 shows an example where red blood cells were stored at 25°C for a period of 14 days. Assuming that one day storage at 25°C is equivalent to one week at 4°C, the usage of such an in-line filter would lead to the possibility of lengthening the storage time of RCCs to up to 14 weeks with maintenance of full function and cell survival.

The main advantages of this concept are not only the potential for a longer storage time (with the possibility of a second anti-HIV test of the donor) but also better quality red cells at any point during the preservation of the product compared to current red cell preservations in existing additive solutions.

In conjunction with the previously addressed concept of haemotherapy, arises the question of the necessary level of leucocyte depletion. This question only can be accurately answered when the critical levels for the stipulated side effects are known. Most probably the currently available log 4 filters are sufficient to prevent alloimmunisation and CMV transmission. However, exceptionally efficient WBC reduction, up to log 6-7, will be necessary to prevent immunosuppressive effects, increased tumour progression and proliferation, and perhaps GVHD, only by the use of filtration.

Figure 5 *Changes in intra-cellular ATP and 2,3-DPG and in chloride ion concentration in the supernatant, presented as percentages of the initial values. In addition, extra- and intracellular pH (pHe, pHi) are shown on the right axis. All RBCs have been white cell- and chloride ion depleted using an experimental in-line filter (DEAE-Cellulose) and were subsequently stored over a period of 15 days at 25°C in a preservation solution containing phosphate, citrate and adenine*

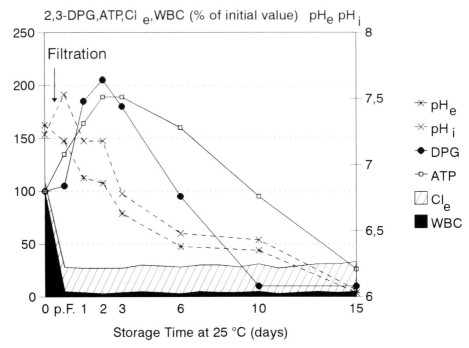

Surely one can foresee that all known data and the findings presented here on the effects of in-line filtration, will lead in the next years, to leucocyte depletion of all red cell concentrates prior to hypothermic storage. This will mean added cost in the preparation of red cell concentrates, but because of the advantages of in-line filtration and considering the subsequent therapy costs which result from the use of non-filtered blood, this will be more than justified.

References

Hau F. (1993) Effect of leukocyte depletion on preservation of erythrocyte and platelet concentrates, *Rev. Fr. Transf. Hemobiol.* 36: 297-304.

Klapper E.B., Goldfinger D. (1992) Leukocyte-reduced blood components in transfusion medicine - Current indications and prospects for the future, *Clin. Lab. Med.* 12: 711-721.

Klein H.G. (1992) Wolf in wolf's clothing: Is it time to raise the bounty on the passenger leuko-cyte?, *Blood* 80: 1865-1867.

Matthes G., Krause K.P., Richter E. (1993a) Verfahren zur Stabilisierung und Rejuvenierung der Sauerstofftransportfähigkeit von konservierten roten Blutzellen. Erfindungsanmeldung P 43 26 713.0, Deutsches Patentamt.

Matthes G., Strunk S., Siems W., Grune T. (1993b) Posttransfusional changes of 2,3-diphospho-glycerate and nucleotides in CPD-SAGM-preserved erythrocytes, *Z. Infusionsther. Transfusionsmed.* 20: 89-92.

Matthes G., Mavrina L., Loth F. (1993b) Verfahren und Filtermaterial zur Stabilisierung und Langzeitkonservierung von roten Blutzellen. Erfindungsanmeldung P 43 31 388.4, Deutsches Patentamt.

Meryman H.T., Hornblower M., Keegan, T. (1991) Refrigerated storage of washed red cells, *Vox Sang.* 60: 88-98

Müller N., Richter E., Matthes G., Kadar J.G. (1993) In-line Filtration mittels Sepacell Integra-System, *Z. Infusionsther. Transfusionsmed.*, in press.

Cost Effectiveness of Leucocyte Depletion

15 | B. Brozović

The majority of patients who receive only once red cells or platelet concentrates (PC) suffer no demonstrable adverse effects from allogeneic 'passenger' leucocytes. Patients who repeatedly receive transfusions may suffer from one or several adverse consequences caused by allogeneic leucocytes (Table 1). Only in a few carefully defined groups of patients a benefit from transfused allogeneic leucocytes can be demonstrated (Mowbray et al. 1987, Silvis et al. 1994).

Table 1 *Adverse consequences which may occur following the transfusion of allogeneic leucocytes*

Alloimmunisation against HLA antigens[1]
    Non-haemolytic febrile transfusion reaction (in patients receiving multiple red cell transfusions)
    Platelet refractoriness (in patients receiving multiple platelet transfusions)
    Rejection of transplanted tissues or solid organs (bone marrow, kidney)

Immunomodulation
    Increased susceptibility to infection (e.g. postoperatively)
    Diminished resistance to cancer recurrence (e.g. postoperatively)

Graft versus host disease
    In immunocompromised patients
    In immunocompetent patients

Reperfusion injury
    In patients undergoing open heart surgery

Transmission of viruses (resident in leucocytes)
    Cytomegalovirus (CMV)[1]
    Epstein-Barr virus (EBV)
    Human immunodeficiency virus (HIV) type 1 and 2[2]
    Human T-cell leukaemia virus (HTLV) type I and II
    Human herpes virus 6 (HHV6)
    JC virus
    BK virus?

1. Documented prevention by transfusion of leucodepleted red cells and cellular blood components with leucocytes content of less than 5×10^6.
2. Transmitted by blood and all non-cellular blood components.

The removal of leucocytes from red cells or PC to less than 5×10^6 will invariably prevent non-haemolytic febrile transfusion reactions (NHFTR) in a immunised recipient. It will also prevent or delay alloimmunisation against HLA antigens and will prevent transmission of cytomegalovirus (CMV). However, it will be of limited or no value in preventing other unwanted consequences. However, leucodepletion is costly and where carried out within cost-conscious health care environment its cost has to be estimated and its benefit to the patient evaluated so that an informed decision on its application can be agreed by health care purchasers and providers. The analysis of cost is a part of the statistical decision theory, and provides information for the decision making process; it comprises calculating cost efficiency, estimating cost effectiveness and evaluating cost benefit (Table 2). Calculating the cost efficiency of leucodepletion is comparatively easy. Estimating cost effectiveness is more difficult as it depends on availability of leucodepleted blood components, numbers of patients requiring leucodepleted components, the local (unit or hospital) policies, and the preferences of the prescribing physician. Evaluating cost benefit, in my view, is not possible at present, because of the absence of measures for clinical outcome on the one hand, and scarcity of data indicating health benefits to patients who had received leucodepleted red cells or PC (also see Perkins 1993, Strauss 1993).

Table 2 *Analysis of cost*

Cost efficiency
    Definition:
    Produce same number of items for less cost or more items for same cost.
    Examples:
    A. Move filtration from the laboratory to the bed side where it is carried out by
        nurses within their 'unoccupied' time (save on labour costs).
    B. Use one filter (intended for one unit) for two units of red cells.

Cost effectiveness
    Definition:
    Achieve the same objective, without loss of quality, using a less expensive alternative
    procedure.
    Example:
    Obtain leucocyte depleted platelet concentrate by cell separator instead of filtered
    pooled random donor platelet concentrates.

Cost benefit
    Definition:
    Quantify the health benefit from a given procedure.
    Example:
    Estimate the extended life expectancy by preventing immunomodulation in a preterm low birth weight baby receiving leucodepleted red cells.

In this presentation the attention will be focused on the factors influencing the estimate of cost effectiveness of leucodepletion with the purpose to demonstrate that the degree of existing variability is sufficient to preclude meaningful comparison of different sets of data.

Leucodepleted red cells and platelet concentrates

The cost of leucodepletion comprises the price of the product, cost of leucodepletion procedure (costs of disposables and labour) and overheads. The costing should be carried out separately for red cells and PC.

The price of a unit of red cells depends on the type of product and complexity of processing (whole blood, red cells in optimal additive solution, red cells buffy coat removed, etc). Only filtration using leucocyte depletion filters with polyester fibres, either native or with a modified surface, will reduce the leucocyte content to below 5×10^6 leucocytes (Table 3). While the price of red cells and the cost of filters are comparable in different hospitals and even in different countries, the labour costs and overheads are highly variable as the filtration can be carried out in regional transfusion centres, hospital blood banks or, quite successfully, on the wards (Sirchia et al. 1994). The costing exercise must take into account occurrence of filter failures and the cost of their consequences as for example when filtering HbAS red cells (Brozovic 1993).

Table 3 *Mean leucocyte content of non-filtered and filtered red cells and platelet concentrates*

Component	Mean leucocyte content per unit	
	Non-filtered	Filtered
Red cells	2.5×10^9	2.5×10^6
Red cells buffy coat removed	5×10^8	$< 10^6$
Random donor platelet concentrate[1]		
PRP method	5×10^8	5×10^6
Buffy coat method	$< 10^7$	$< 10^5$
Single donor platelet concentrate, plateletpheresis[2]	5×10^6	$< 10^5$

1. Six units or a pool equivalent to six units.
2. Using Spectra (COBE), CS-3000 Plus (Baxter) with TNX-6 or AS104 (Fresenius cell separator)

There are two different ways to obtain an adult platelet dose (absolute number of platelets higher than 3×10^{11}) with the leucocyte count if less than 5×10^6. The first one is to filter single units or pooled PC prepared from random donors, and the second one is to collect platelets using a Spectra (COBE), CS-3000 Plus (Baxter) or AS104 (Fresenius) or similar cell separator. In the latter instance the capital and revenue costs as well as overheads vary so much from one site to another that it is unlikely that a valid costing comparison could ever be made.

Routine leucocyte depletion of red cells will increase the safety of blood components with respect to transmission of bacteria, providing that the filtration is carried out within the period from 5 to 24 hours after blood collection (Högman 1991, 1992).

It is of interest that recent observations have indicated that not all transfusion reactions are prevented by administration of leucodepleted red cells (Mangano et al. 1991). The transfusion reactions, seen particularly in recipients of PC, have been associated with high levels of interleukin 6 (IL-6) and tumour necrosis factor α (TNFα) in the plasma (Muylle et al. 1993). These reactions should not be considered as filtration failures but should be assessed as matters of quality related to the prolonged storage of PC.

Patients

There is a general agreement that administration of leucodepleted red cells (less than 5×10^6 leucocytes) and/or PC is recommended in the following groups of patients (Consensus Conference 1993):

- transfusion dependent patients who receive red cells and have recurrent NHFTR or in whom the prevention of immunisation is intended
- newly diagnosed patients with aplastic anaemia who are potential recipients of bone marrow transplants
- pregnant women receiving intrauterine transfusions of cellular blood components
- immuno-incompetent CMV seronegative patients when CMV antibody-negative cellular components are not available

Possible indications for leucocyte depletion of blood components are aimed at preventing adverse effects of allogeneic leucocytes listed in Table 1 in a variety of patients (for details see Consensus Conference 1993).

Evaluation of cost effectiveness of leucodepletion in each patient group has been limited by the diversity of criteria for inclusion of patients into the study groups and by the lack of definitions for outcome measures. These problems were analysed in detail by Heddle (1994) in her critical appraisal of the efficacy of leucodepletion to improve platelet transfusion response. Nevertheless, it has been possible to identify three sets of factors which have to be taken into account when evaluating cost effectiveness of leucodepletion aimed to prevent immunisation against HLA antigens.

First, it has been demonstrated that patients who posses DRw2 HLA antigen have on average twice the chance to develop platelet refractoriness (Brand et al. 1989). Thus an inherited phenotype may influence the clinical outcome of a policy on administration of leucodepleted products.

Secondly, it has been demonstrated that parous women develop more readily platelet refractoriness than those without children or men (Brand et al. 1989). Furthermore, it has been shown in a prospective study that administration of leucocyte depleted single donor PC does not prevent secondary HLA alloimmunisation and platelet refractoriness (Sintnicolaas et al. 1994). Those observations illustrate how factors acquired earlier in life affect the clinical outcome, and in turn, evaluation of cost effectiveness.

Finally, in a clinical setting, there has been no general agreement on the concentration of platelets in the patient below which a transfusion of platelets is deemed necessary (Beutler 1993). In addition, the use of the platelet count following transfusion as a measure of clinical outcome, even where expressed as corrected count index (CCI) leaves much to be desired. New tests, such as the 'in vitro bleeding time' described by Högman et al. (1993) still await testing in the field. Invariably the analysis of the clinical outcome should involve the follow up of the recipient to reveal beneficial effects of transfusion of leucodepleted blood components which may become apparent only after some time. In a retrospective study on 115 patients with acute myeloid leukaemia Oksanen and Elonen (1993) have demonstrated that there were no differences in the clinical presentation of patients who received leucocyte depleted blood components and those who did not during the first cycle of treatment. However, during subsequent treatment periods in the former group of patients the requirement for red cells and PC was significantly smaller, granulocytopenia (less than 0.5×10^9/L) and thrombocytopenia (less than 50×10^9/L) were shorter, serious infections were less common and the patients spent fewer days in hospital. Perhaps the most important finding was that the median relapse-free survival was longer in the patients receiving leucodepleted blood components. These observations highlight the need for follow-up of patients over a prolonged period of time.

The diversity of patients receiving leucodepleted blood components, no defined clinical outcome, and a time lag required for manifestation of some of the effects following transfusion of allogeneic leucocytes makes it impossible to evaluate cost effectiveness of leucodepletion.

The way forward

The way forward in providing realistic and reliable cost effectiveness analysis requires the establishment of sound costing and pricing mechanisms and agreeing on the measures of the clinical outcome in patients receiving multiple transfusion of red cells and PC. That would allow comparisons between studies performed at different centres and would also enable both the clinicians and managers to design an appropriate model for cost benefit analysis, which has been and still remains an elusive target.

References

Beutler E. (1993) Platelet transfusions: the 20,000/μL trigger, *Blood* 81: 1411-1413.
Brand A. Claas F.H.J., Gratama J.W., Eermisse J.G. (1989) Leucocyte-depleted blood components prevent primary HLA immunization in the majority of patients receiving multiple blood transfusions, in: Brozovic B. (ed.) *The Role of Leucocyte Depletion in Blood Transfusion Practice*, Blackwell Scientific Publications, Oxford, pp. 4-7.

Brozovic B. (1993) Leukocyte depletion of blood and blood components: current problems and solutions, in: Sekigudri S. (ed.) *Clinical Application of Leucocyte Depletion*, Blackwell Scientific Publication, Oxford, pp. 223-230.

Consensus conference (1993) *Leucocyte Depletion of Blood and Blood Components*, The Royal College of Physicians, Edinburgh.

Heddle N.M. (1994) The efficacy of leukodepletion to improve platelet transfusion response: a critical appraisal of clinical studies, *Transfusion Med. Rev.* 8: 15-28.

Högman C.F., Eriksson L., Kristensen J. (1993) Leucocyte-depleted platelets prepared from pooled buffy coat post-transfusion increment are 'in vitro bleeding time' using the thrombostat 4000/2, *Transf. Sci.* 14: 35-39.

Högman C.F., Gong J., Eriksson L., Hambraeus A., Johansson C.S. (1991) White cell protect donor blood against bacterial contamination, *Transfusion* 31: 620-626.

Högman C.F., Gong J., Hambraeus A., Johansson C.S., Eriksson L. (1992) The role of white cells in the transmission of Yersinia enterocolitica in blood components, *Transfusion* 32: 654-657.

Mangano M.M., Chamber L.A., Kruskall M.S. (1991) Limited efficiency of leukopoor platelets for prevention of febrile transfusion reactions, *Am. J. Clin. Pathol.* 95: 733-738.

Mowbray J.F., Underwood J.C., Michel M., Forbes P.R., Beard R.W. (1987) Immunization with paternal lymphocytes in women with recurrent spontaneous abortion, *Lancet* ii: 679-680.

Muylle L., Joos M., Wouters E., De Bock R., Peetermans M.E. (1993) Increased tumor necrosis factor α (TBFα), interleukin 1, and interleukin 6 (IL-6) levels in the plasma of stored platelet concentrates: relationship between TNFα and IL-6 levels and febrile transfusion reactions, *Transfusion*, 33: 195-199.

Oksanen K., Elonen E. (1993) Impact of leucocyte-depleted blood components on the haematological recovery and prognosis of patients with acute myeloid leukaemia, *Bri. J. Haematol.* 84: 639-647.

Perkins H.A. (1993) Is white cell reduction cost-effective?, *Transfusion* 33: 626-628.

Silvis R., Steup W.H., Brand A., Zwinderman K.A.H., Lamers C.B.H.W., Griffioen G., Gooszen H.G. (1994) Protective effect of blood transfusions on preoperative recurrence of Crohn's disease in parous women, *Transfusion* 34: 242-247.

Sintnicolaas K., Van Marwijk Kooij M., Van Prooijen H.C., Van Dijk B.A., Van Putten W.L.J., Novotny V.M.J., Brand A. (1994) Leukocyte depletion of random single donor platelet transfusions does not prevent secondary HLA-alloimmunization and refractoriness: a randomised prospective study, *Abstracts of the XIII Congress of the International Society of Blood Transfusion*, Amsterdam.

Sirchia G., Rebulla P., Parravicini A., Marangoni F., Cortelezzi A., Stefania A. (1994) Quality control of red cell filtration at the patient's bedside, *Transfusion* 34: 26-30.

Strauss R.G. (1993) Selection of white cell-reduced blood components for transfusion during early infancy, *Transfusion* 33: 353-357.

Comparison Between Nageotte Hemocytometer and Flow Cytometer Counting Methods for the Detection of Residual Leucocytes in Plateletapheresis Products

H.S.P. Garritsen, P. Krakowitzky, K. Härtel, K. Lippert, F. Smeets, C. Schneider and W. Sibrowski

16

Introduction

The accurate detection and counting on a routine basis, of contaminating leucocytes in plateletapheresis products, remains a problem in transfusion medicine. The range of leucocyte contamination is in general believed to be $< 10^7$ leucocytes/apheresis product (240-300 ml). This is below the limit of accurate detection using automated methods for counting leucocytes (Friedman et al. 1990, Dumont 1991).

Microscopic evaluation of leucocyte contamination (Nageotte chamber) is not suitable for counting leucocyte contamination on a routine basis, therefore several alternative techniques (Kao and Scornik 1989, Bodensteiner 1989, Dzik et al. 1990, Stienstra and Vos 1991), including quantitative PCR (Abe et al. 1993) have been proposed.

We evaluated a flow cytometric method (FCM) using fluorescent microspheres and compared these results with the results of microscopic evaluation (Nageotte hemocytometer) in 23 samples from plateletapheresis products. A good correlation between FCM and microscopic evaluation could be obtained (r = 0.8918). The accurate determination of the concentration of the fluorescent microspheres turned out to be an important issue.

Material and methods

Material
Apheresis platelets were prepared at our cytapheresis unit, from healthy donors, using the Cobe Spectra (Cobe Laboratories, Munich, Germany) and the AS 104 (Fresenius, Oberursel, Germany).

Microscopic evaluation
Manual counting of leucocytes present in platelet concentrates was done using a modified Nageotte chamber. The platelet sample was first diluted 5 fold in

'Türks' solution. Platelet suspensions were incubated in the diluent for 10 minutes at room temperature and then 75 μl aliquots were pipetted onto the hemocytometer equipped with a cover slip. This sample was allowed to settle undisturbed for 10 minutes at room temperature in a moist petri dish to prevent evaporation. The hemocytometer was then examined under a phase contrast microscope (x16) and the leucocytes present in one grid were counted. This is 50 μl of diluted platelet suspension.

Flow cytometry

The samples for FCM were prepared according to Dzik et al. (1990) with the modification that fluorescent microspheres were added. Briefly 200μl of platelet sample was added to 1000μl of propidium iodide solution. Subsequently 10μl of fluorescent microspheres (red fluorescent CaliBrite beads, Becton Dickinson, San Jose, Cal.) with known concentration were added . The mixture was allowed to incubate at room temperature for 15 minutes before flow cytometric analysis. The microsphere-cell suspension was analysed using a FACScan flow cytometer operating at 488nm, at 15 mW power, using Lysis II software (BDIS). Data were acquired of 5,000 gated events. Gating was performed on right angle light scattering and propidium iodide fluorescence in FL2 (red fluorescence). The fluorescence channels were set at logarithmic gain.

Calculation of the leucocyte concentration for:

Nageotte Chamber:

$$WBC/\mu l = \frac{Number\ of\ WBC\ per\ grid}{10}$$

Flow cytometry:

$$WBC/\mu l = \frac{\%\ of\ PI\ WBC\ nuclei\ events}{\%\ of\ fl.\ microspheres} \times \frac{total\ number\ fl.\ microspheres}{200}$$

PI: propidium iodide
WBC: white blood cells

Statistics

Pearson's co-efficient of correlation was used to investigate the univariate relationship between FCM and microscopic evaluation. Because of the large range in WBC counts (0-307.69/μl) and the highly skewed distributions of both methods, we decided to make a logarithmic transformation of the results. Values of Spearman correlation on the original results were not different from results of Pearson correlation of the transformed values.

Results

Figure 1 and 2 show the two-parameter dot-plots of side scatter vs. forward scatter (Figure 1) and side scatter vs. FL2 (propidium iodide) respectively. In Figure 1 the microspheres are easily detected and distinguished from other events due to their low forward scatter and relatively high side scatter characteristics.

In Figure 2 the propidium iodide labelled leucocytes are easily distinguished from other events due to their high propidium iodide uptake. Again the microspheres can be discriminated on the basis of side scatter characteristics.

Figure 1 *A two-parameter dot plot of scatter parameters (FSC: forward scatter, SSC: side scatter) of a sample, containing relatively high numbers of WBCs*

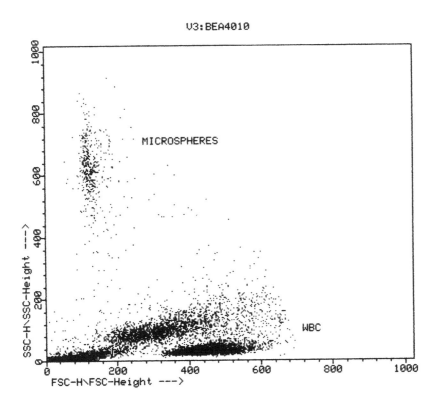

Figure 2 *Two-parameter dot-plot of fluoresence-channel 2 and* SSC *of the same sample*

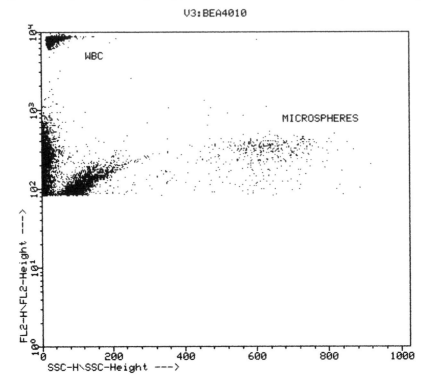

U3:BEA4010

Data were analysed by setting analysing gates around the regions of interest (WBC and microspheres). The percentages of events falling in one of these regions were used to calculate the concentration of leucocytes in plateletapheresis products as described in material and methods.

Figure 3 displays the results of the comparison of leucocyte contamination of 23 samples from plateletapheresis products. Nageotte chamber counting was compared with the proposed FCM method.

The correlation between FCM and microscopic evaluation is high (0.8918) and clearly significant (p=0.0001). Spread of variability, as measured by the coefficient of variation, was higher for FCM (140.7%) than for the microscopic evaluation (97.2%)

Discussion

For counting very low levels of leucocytes a number of different methods are available (Kao and Scornik 1989, Bodensteinder 1989, Dzik et al. 1990, Stienstra and Vos 1991, Abe et al. 1993). Although the Nageotte chamber (Wenz et al. 1991) is recognised as approaching a 'gold standard' for leucocyte counting, the microscopic counting is time consuming and the accurate identification of cell types can be difficult. These considerations have limited the use of the Nageotte chamber to scientific studies and prevented its use as a routine method in the quality control of platelet concentrates in most institutes for blood transfusion. Flow cytometry has been proposed as an alternative method for counting very low levels of leucocytes in blood components. The discrimination of leucocytes from erythrocytes or platelets is mostly achieved by using a specific fluorescent DNA-stain (Bodensteiner 1989, Dzik et al. 1990) which can be excited at 488nm and has a maximum emission around 530nm or around 580nm.

Figure 3 *The concentration of WBCs measured by Nageotte chamber is plotted as a function of the WBC concentration as determined by FCM. Correlation coefficient r = 0.8918*

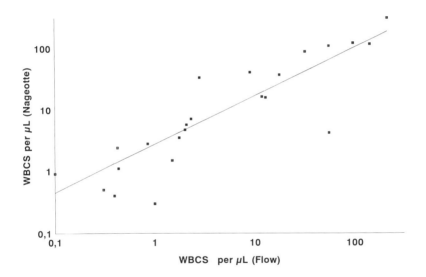

Stienstra and de Vos (Stienstra and Vos 1991) already showed that it is possible to identify leucocytes in platelet concentrates solely on the basis of their scatter properties by manipulating the scatter properties of the platelets using a specific preparation procedure.

In our view the scatter properties of events only, are not enough to define cells as leucocytes. We therefore developed a flow cytometric method which is a modification of the method of Dzik et al. (1990) and which uses the ratio of fluorescent beads (with known concentration) to leucocytes (defined by propidium iodide staining) to determine the concentration of the leucocytes. Fluorescent beads were chosen instead of fluorescein-labelled chicken red cells (see Vachula et al. 1993) because of their stability. The determination of the concentration of beads was done by microscopic counting and became an important issue with respect to the variability of the results.

In future studies we plan to do the determination of the microsphere concentration by an automatic counter. The FCM time needed to acquire the data, after sample preparation, was 10 minutes. In general FCM seems to be a favourable alternative to Nageotte chamber counting for routine quality control for several reasons. There is a good correlation between FCM and Nageotte chamber counting, FCM is more or less independent of the concentration of the technician who can only perform a limited number of Nageotte chamber countings. FCM measurements did not take as much time as Nageotte chamber measurements.

Therefore we believe that this FCM method is well suited for routine quality control and the detection of residual leucocyte levels in plateletapheresis products.

References

Abe H., Hosoda M., Takahashi T. A., Sekiguchi S. (1993) Polymerase chain reaction method for counting extremely low numbers of leucocytes in blood products prepared with 6 log leucocyte removal filters (Abstract S13) '46th Meeting American Association of Blood Bankers Miami', 23-29 October.

Bodensteiner D.C. (1989) A flow cytometric technique to accurately measure post-filtration white blood cellcounts, *Transfusion* 29: 651-653.

Dumont L.J. (1991) Sampling errors and the precision associated with counting very low numbers of white cells in blood components, *Transfusion* 31: 428-432.

Dzik W.H., Ragosta A., Cusack W. (1990) Flow cytometric method for counting very low numbers of leucocytes in platelets products, *Vox Sang.* 59: 153-159.

Friedman L.I., Sadoff B.J., Stromberg R.R. (1990) White cell counting in red cells and platelets: how few can we count?, *Transfusion* 30: 387-389.

Kao K., Scornik J. (1989) Accurate quantification of the low number of white cells in white cell depleted blood components, *Transfusion* 29: 774-777.

Stienstra S., De Vos D. (1991) Quality control of leukocyte depletion in bloodbanking with a flow cytometer:flow cytometry to determine low concentration of white cells in leukocyte-poor platelet concentrates, in: Sekiguchi S. (ed.) *Clinical Application of Leukocyte Depletion, Proceedings of the 3rd Hokkaido Symposium on Transfusion Medicine 1991*, Blackwell Scientific Publications, Oxford, pp. 63-76.

Vachula M., Simpson S.J., Martinson J.A., Aono F.M., Hutchcraft A.M., Balma D.L., Van Epps D.E. (1993) A flow cytometric method for counting very low levels of white cells in blood and blood components, *Transfusion* 33: 262-267.

Wenz B., Burns E., Lee V., Miller W. (1991) A rare event analysis model for quantifying white cells in white cell-depleted blood, *Transfusion* 31: 156-159.

Polymerase Chain Reaction Method to Count Residual Leucocytes in Red Cell Concentrates Prepared with a High-efficiency Leucocyte Removal Filter

17 T.A. Takahashi, H. Abe, M. Hosoda and S. Sekiguchi

Introduction

A high-efficiency leucocyte-removal filter has been introduced experimentally to our laboratory for evaluation. The filter is able to eliminate leucocytes to below the detection limit of flow cytometric (FCM) method (Takahashi et al. 1990) and Cytospin method (Takahashi et al. 1989), which have the highest sensitivity among the current counting methods. We applied a polymerase chain reaction (PCR) method to measure a small number of leucocytes in blood products which were filtered by the filter. A single-copy gene, ß-globin gene, was amplified in the PCR.

Materials and methods

From 400 mL of whole blood routinely donated, red cell concentrates (RCC) were prepared by centrifugation at 4530x g for 6 min and then filtered through the high-efficiency leucocyte-removal filter (Asahi Medical, Tokyo, Japan). FCM method: 100 μL of RCC was mixed with 750 μL of propidium iodide (PI) solution. After 10 min incubation at room temperature, leucocytes were counted by FCM (Cytoron, Ortho). The detection limit of this method was 177 cells/mL. The improved FCM method was performed with the 10-fold concentrated sample, and the detection limit was 17.7 cells/mL (Takahashi et al. 1993). PCR method: RCC was serially 10-fold diluted with Hanks' balanced salt solution (HBSS) and 1 mL of each diluent was hemolyzed and washed with 10 mM Tris-HCL (pH 8.0), 1 mM EDTA, and 10 mM NaCl by centrifugation. The pellet was treated with Proteinase K (Sigma, USA) in the presence of glycogen as a carrier of DNA. After phenol/chloroform extraction, DNA was precipitated with ethanol, washed with 70% ethanol, vacuum desiccated, and dissolved in H_2O. Total DNA extract prepared from 1 mL of sample was applied for PCR. One-step PCR was examined using 25 pmol of GH20 and GH21 oligonucleotide as primers (Takara, Japan) and PC04 oligonucleotide (Takara) as a probe. The reaction was repeated 35 cycles at 94°C for 30 sec, 55°C for 30 sec, and 72°C for 90 sec by a thermal cycler (System

9600, Perkin-Elmer Cetus). The amplified DNA was detected by ^{32}P-labeled PC04 by Southern hybridization. For a non-radioisotopic method, we examined nested-double PCR using 5 pmol of GH20 and GH21 for 1st step and 25 pmol of KM29 and KM38 oligonucleotide (Takara) for 2nd step. The reaction was repeated 25 cycles in the 1st step and 35 cycles in the 2nd step. After PCR, the amplified DNA was analyzed by agarose gel electrophoresis with ethidium bromide staining under UV light.

Results

Using 10-fold dilution series of purified peripheral mononuclear cells in HBSS, one-step PCR showed the detection limit at 2.4 cells in 18 mL. The similar sensitivity was obtained by the nested-double PCR. This detection sensitivity was 10- to 100-fold higher than that obtained by FCM method. We used the nested-double PCR to count the residual leucocytes in RCC filtered through the high-efficiency leucocyte-removal filter. To estimate the concentration of the leucocytes, RCC was serially 10-fold diluted and each diluent was assayed in quintuplicate by PCR. When RCC containing 10^6 cells/mL was diluted, PCR could detect DNA in all the five measurement at 10^{-6} diluent. Further dilution failed to detect DNA in some of five measurement. Therefore, we interpreted that the end-point dilution which gave five positive was the concentration of the leucocytes in original solution.

Table 1 *Leucocyte counts by the improved FCM and nested-double PCR in filtered RCC*

Number of leucocytes (cells/ml)			
Improved FCM		PCR	$(10^0, 10^{-1}, 10^{-2})$
3.5*	(0,0,0,1,0)**	10^0	(5/5, 2/5, 0/5)***
7.1	(0,0,1,0,1)	10^1	(5/5, 5/5, 2/5)
3.5	(0,0,1,0,0)	10^0	(5/5, 0/5, 0/5)
< 3.5	(0,0,0,0,0)	10^1	(5/5, 5/5, 0/5)

* calculated from the average of total events in five measurements
** number of fluorescent events in five each measurements
*** number of PCR positive sample/number of tested samples

The PCR method could detect leucocytes in all the samples of filtered RCC and showed that the numbers of residual leucocytes were in the range of 10^0 to 10^2 cells/mL (see Table 1). On the other hand, the FCM method could not detect leucocytes in many samples.

Discussion

We have developed a non-isotopic PCR method for counting residual leucocytes in the filtered RCC. Hemoglobin is known to inhibit PCR, so the RCC was hemolyzed and washed until the red colour was invisible. We used glycogen, which does not inhibit PCR, as a carrier of DNA to obtain an excellent recovery of very small amount of DNA. No leucocytes were detected by FCM method, meaning that the residual leucocytes were below 177 cells/mL. Although the concentration of leucocytes were calculated to be <3.54 to 7.08 cells/mL from the improved FCM measurement, no cell was detected in many samples in their measurement (Table 1). Virtually, only four events were observed in twenty measurements, and the numbers of residual leucocytes were below the detection limit of the improved FCM method. These results show that the PCR will be useful for the evaluation of the new generation filters and for the quality control of leucocyte-depleted blood products.

References

Takahashi T.A. et al. (1990) A flow cytometric method to detect residual leukocytes in platelet and red cell concentrates, *Jpn. J. Transfus. Med.* 36: 429-437.

Takahashi T.A. et al. (1989) Cytospin method for the determination of residual leukocytes in leukocyte-depleted platelet concentrates, *Jpn. J. Transfus. Med.* 35: 497-503.

Takahashi T.A. et al. (1993) Comparison of highly sensitive methods used to count residual leukocytes in filtered red cell and platelet concentrates, in Sekiguchi S. (ed.) *Clinical Application of Leukocyte Depletion*, Blackwell Scientific Publications, Oxford, pp. 77-91.

Identifications of Different Types of White Blood Cells in Buffy Coat-depleted Red Cell Units Using Flow Cytometry

18 | F. Knutson and C.F. Högman

The leucocyte content in buffy-coat depleted RBC concentrates (SAGM supension) has been identified using flow cytometry. Most of the remaining WBCs were granulocytes (CD45+, CD3-, CD19-). Most units contained less than 5×10^6 MNCs, with decreasing concentration during storage, but examples of clearcut drop-outs were observed.

Introduction

Removal of buffy coat from red blood cell units (RBC) is a commonly used measure to improve their quality. The procedure is more effective with respect to mononuclear cells (MNC) than granulocytes (Nakajo et al. 1993). Using flow cytometry we have identified white blood cells (WBC) in buffy-coat depleted RBC during the first week of refrigerator storage.

Methods

Blood was collected from normal donors, 450 ml of blood in 63 ml CPD solution using the Opti System® (Baxter, Lessines, France). After 4-6 h at 22°C blood components were prepared using the Optipress®, 50-55 ml buffy coat was retained in the original bag (Högman et al. 1988). The RBCs were transferred to a bag with 100 ml SAGM solution and stored at 4°C. Sampling was performed after 16-20 h, 2, 3, 4 and 7 d.

Flow cytometry was used with an Ortho Cytoron Absolute® device (Ortho Diagnostics, Raritan, New Jersey). In a first series of 20 RBC units the proportions of lymphocytes, monocytes and granulocytes were identified morphologically, with respect to their light scattering patterns. In a second series of 15 units they were identified both morphologically and on the basis of antigenic determinants using monoclonal antibodies (MoAbs). The MoAbs used (Ortho Diagnostics) were: CD45(Fitc)/CD14(Pe) identifying panleucocyte and monocyte determinants, respectively, CD19(Fitc)/CD3(Pe) identifying B-cells and T-cells, respectively. 25 μl MoAb diluted 1:5 was added to a 100 μl sample and incubated for 15 min in darkness; 2 ml of Ortho-mune Lysing Reagent were added after mixing, incubated for 10 min and washed once with PBS.

On a basis of light-scattering properties, each cell is represented by a point in a rectangular coordinate system (Figure 1). According to the place of the cluster in the whole blood, discrimination frames were placed around MNC and lymphocytes.

Figure 1 *Light scattering patterns of WBCs in whole blood (WB, left) and buffy-coat depleted red cell SAGM suspension (right), showing effective removal of lymphocytes (lower left in WB) and monocytes (upper left in WB)*

FSC

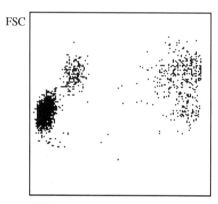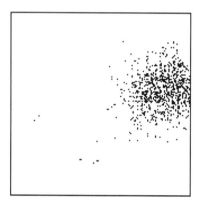

SSC

Results and discussion

The number of remaining MNC in the first series was 3.96×10^6 (range <0.3-21.7×10^6/unit). About 75% of the units contained $<5 \times 10^6$ cells. The majority of remaining WBCs were granulocytes as shown in Figure 1. Figure 2 demonstrates that light scattering as well as MoAb binding properties' changes during 7-day storage.

Table 1 *Presence of mononuclear cells in buffy coat reduced red cell concentrates, $x10^6/l$, mean $\pm 1SD$*

	No. of MNC	No. of lymphocytes	No. of CD3	No. of CD19
Day 1	11.2±4.3	4.2±3.2	1.5±1.2	0.3±0.5
Day 2	14.0±8.5	2.7±2.1	0.7±0.7	0.2±0.4
Day 3	12.6±5.8	4.0±2.3	1.2±0.8	0.5±0.5
Day 4	9.8±6.2	3.6±3.4	0.1±0.1	0.012±0.022
Day 7	4.9±3.2	0.8±0.9	0.4±0.4	0.041±0.083

The number of MNCs identified according to their site in the light scattering diagram were 11-14x10^6 during the first three days and then decreased (Table 1). The number of lymphocytes (x10^6/l) identifiable with MoAbs was about 1.5 (T-cells) and 0.3 (B-cells) but 4.2 as judged from light scattering. A decrease was seen during storage. In one out of the 15 units in series 2 (figures not included in Table 1) leucocyte reduction after buffy coat removal was very poor, 2,1x10^9 WBCs. In this case the MNC content was 58x10^6, CD3+ 32x10^6 and CD19+ 1.5x10^6. Lymphocytes were still detected after 2 weeks.

We conclude that in the majority of buffy coat-depleted RBC units most of the remaining WBCs were granulocytes and less than 5x10^6 were MNCs. However examples of large numbers of MNCs were found when the leucocyte reducing procedure had been ineffective. The technique described seems to be useful in the validation of blood component quality.

Figure 2 Light scattering pattern of granulocytes (upper part of figure), size (FSC) vs granulation (SSC) showing a change during storage, and CD45 positive cells (lower part of figure) showing lower fluorescence intensity after 7 days

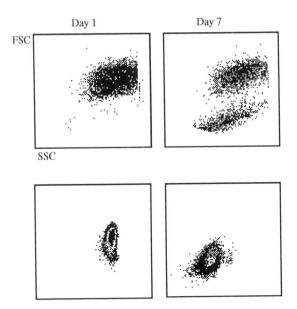

References

Högman C.F., Eriksson L., Hedlund K., Wallvik J. (1988) The bottom and top system: a new technique for blood component preparation and storage, *Vox Sang.* 55: 211-217.

Nakajo S., Chiba S., Takahashi T.A., Sekiguchi S. (1993) Comparison of a 'top and bottom' system with a conventional quadruple-bag system for blood-component preparation and storage, in: Sekiguchi S. (ed.) *Clinical Application of Leukocyte Depletion*, Blackwell Scientific Publications, Oxford, pp. 18-30.

Cooling and Warming Method for Preparation of 1 log Leucocyte-removed Red Cell Concentrates Using the Top & Bottom System

T.A. Takahashi, S. Nakajo, S. Chiba, M. Hosoda and
S. Sekiguchi

19

Introduction

The number of leucocytes in buffy coat-poor red cell concentrate (BPRCC) prepared by the top and bottom system is significantly lower than that prepared by the conventional system. However, the removal rate of leucocytes still remains 70-80% (Nakajo et al., 1993). Most of the residual leucocytes were granulocytes. The population of lymphocytes and monocytes in residual leucocytes is less than 0.05% of the total leucocytes and their number is less than $1x10^6$ cells/bag. We developed a method which can remove 90% of whole blood leucocytes in BPRCC while maintaining high removal rates of lymphocytes and monocytes.

Materials and methods

1. *Preparation of blood components*
    Whole blood (400 mL) was collected in a top and bottom bag (Kawasumi-Baxter). Before centrifugation, a whole blood was stored as follows.
    Standard Method:
        stored at room temperature for 4 hrs.
    Cooling Method:
        stored at 4°C in a cold room for 1, 4, 15 or 24 h.
    Cooling and Warming Method:
        stored at 4°C in a cold room for 4, 15 or 24 h, warmed to 25°C in a water bath for 30 min.
    Rapid Cooling and Warming Method:
        stored at 4°C in a water bath for 4 h, then warmed to 25°C in a water bath for 30 min.

Whole blood was centrifuged at 2560 g for 10 min at 22°C. BPRCC (additive solution: MAP) and platelet-poor plasma (PPP) were prepared using a semi-automated component extractor (Optipress; Baxter).

2. *Counting method*

The number of cells and hematocrit value were counted and measured by the Coulter Counter S-Plus IV. The subpopulations of leucocytes in BPRCC were determined by the cytospin method.

3. *Laboratory testing*

[Red cells] ATP and 2, 3-DPG:UV, Plasma-free hemoglobin: Fluorene, Osmotic fragility: Coil Planet Centrifuge [Plasma] Factor VIII coagulation activity: APTT, Factor VIII associated antigen: EIA.

Results

1. *Characterization of blood components prepared by the cooling method and by the cooling and warming method*

a. Cooling method

When whole blood was stored at 4°C in a cold room for 1 h prior to the centrifugation, the removal rate of total leucocytes and granulocytes in BPRCC were higher than in those prepared by the standard method.

The removal rates of lymphocytes and monocytes, and the recovery rate of red cells were well maintained. However, when whole blood was stored at 4°C for longer than 1 h, the removal rate of leucocytes, particularly lymphocytes in BPRCC decreased. The volume of plasma prepared by the cooling method was significantly lower than those prepared by the standard method.

b. Cooling and Warming Method

The removal rates of total leucocyte, lymphocyte, monocyte and granulocyte in BPRCC prepared by the cooling and warming method were higher than those prepared by the cooling method. The recovery rate of plasma in PPP prepared by the cooling and warming method was also higher than that prepared by the cooling method.

2. *Comparison of characteristics of blood components prepared by the standard method and by the rapid cooling and warming method*

The removal rate of leucocytes in BPRCC prepared by the rapid cooling and warming method was $91.4 \pm 5.2\%$ (Table 1). It was significantly higher than that prepared by the standard method ($p < 0.001$). There was no difference in the recovery rate of red cells and the removal rate of lymphocytes in BPRCC. The recovery rate of plasma in PPP was not different between the two methods.

3. *Condition of red cells in BPRCC*

The condition of red cells in BPRCC prepared by the rapid cooling and warming method was maintained for up to 6 weeks as well as those prepared by the standard method.

4. *Factor VIII activities in PPP*

There was no difference in the factor VIII activity in PPP prepared whether by the standard method or by the rapid cooling and warming method.

Table 1

Components	Standard	Rapid Cooling and Warming
BPRCC		
Volume (ml)	269.9±12.9	281.6±15.3
Hematocrit value (%)	58.0±2.4	58.6±2.0
Leucocyte (x10⁸)	5.53±3.16	2.34±1.38
removal rate (%)	78.3±11.0*	91.4±5.2*
Lymphocyte (x10⁶)	< 0.98	< 0.49
removal rate (%)	> 99.86	> 99.95
Monocyte (x10⁶)	< 0.98	< 0.49
removal rate (%)	> 99.5	> 99.3
Granulocyte (x10⁸)	5.52±3.16	2.34±1.37
removal rate (%)	60.9±18.8*	84.2±9.6*
Red cell (x10¹²)	1.73±0.14	1.83±0.16
recovery rate (%)	86.3±2.6	87.5±4.7
PPP		
Volume (ml)	251.4±12.0	242.1±3.1
recovery rate (%)	86.1±1.2	84.9±3.1

* $P < 0.001$, n=20, mean±1 SD

Discussion and conclusion

Nearly 1 log of leucocyte-depleted BPRCC could be prepared by the top and bottom system if the whole blood was cooled and warmed before centrifugation. When whole blood was stored at 4°C in a water bath for 4 hrs and then warmed to 25°C in a water bath for 30 min before centrifugation, the removal rate of leucocytes in BPRCC was 91.4±5.2%. The number of residual lymphocytes was less than 1x10⁶ cells/bag. Cooling and warming procedures did not affect the biochemical functions of red cells and the qualities of Factor VIII.

These results indicate that the cooling and warming treatment of the whole blood before centrifugation make it possible to deplete 90% of leucocytes when the top and bottom system is used for preparation of blood components.

Reference

Nakajo et al. (1993) Comparison of a 'Top and Bottom' system with a conventional quadruple-bag system for blood component preparation and storage, in Sekiguchi S. (ed.) *Clinical Application of Leukocyte Depletion*, Blackwell Scientific Publications, Oxford, pp. 18-30.

Leucocyte Depletion in Blood Transfusion and Survival After Radical Surgery for Malignant Tumours

20 | E. Haglind

In the last decade a number of studies have reported increased 5-year survival in patients who did not receive blood transfusion at radical surgery for malignant tumours as compared to patients who did receive blood transfusion. These studies were all retrospective in nature and did not aim to determine what factor, if any, in blood transfusions that could play a role for long term survival (Salo 1988).

Early observations on the possible immunosuppressive effect of blood transfusions were reported by Opelz and co-workers, when they found increased transplant survival after kidney transplantation in patients who had previously received blood transfusions (Opelz et al. 1973).

Transfusion of leucocytes have been found to trigger antibody production in the recipient, resulting in antibodies blocking several different cellular immunoreactions in the recipient (Unander 1992). The aim of the present study is to determine the effect on survival in two groups of patients: the control group receiving traditional blood products and the test group receiving leucocyte depleted blood products after radical surgery for malignant tumours.

Material and method:
The study is a prospective, randomised, multicentre study

Inclusion criteria
Patients undergoing radical surgery for malignant tumours in the GI-tract and the kidney. Patients are excluded when the operation is not considered to be radical. Surgery is considered to be radical when no distant metastases are found and when the surgeon considers that he has performed local radical surgery at operation. No special preoperative routines to detect distant metastases have been part of the study protocol. Thus the routines in each participating Department of Surgery have been continued without change.

Randomisation
Patients included in the protocol are randomised preoperatively to one group receiving traditional blood products (control) and one group (the test group) receiving leucocyte depleted blood products. Randomisation is by a date of birth. Patients who do not need transfusion during operation will be part of an observa-

tion group, that is comparable to the non-transfused groups of the retrospective studies. This group is not strictly part of the protocol but will be followed in the same manner as the test and the control groups.

Study design
The study is designed as a multicentre study and the participating Departments of Surgery have been recruited from Sahlgrens University Hospital, Göteborg; Mölndal Hospital, Kungälv Hospital, Borås Hospital, Alingsås Hospital and Lidköping Hospital. Inclusion of patients started in Sahlgrens University Hospital in 1990 and gradually the study was then started in the other participating hospitals.

Filter technique
Depletion of leucocytes has been by Sepacell filter in the test group. All erythrocyte and plasma products are filtered.

Study end point
The end point of the study is the 5-year survival rate in the two groups. In order to show a 20% difference in survival rate with a 95% confidence limit, the study has to include 650 patients.

Patient follow-up will be by routines ordinarily used in each hospital. The 5-year survival rate will be analysed through the Swedish Death Register in combination with the Swedish Cancer Register.

Results

Up to March 1st, 1994 the total of of 786 patients have been included in the study. The transfusion rate has been constant at 60% during the three years of inclusion.

Colorectal cancer is the largest group with 537 patients followed by renal cancer with 104. The median number of transfused units in the test group was 2.2 and in the control group 2.7. The number of plasma units given were correspondingly 1.4 and 2.6. There is no difference in median age between the test and control group. The distribution of colorectal cancers according to the Dukes classification is the same in both test and control groups.

Summary

We report on a prospective, randomised trial of leucocyte depleted transfusion products and their effect on long term survival after radical surgery for malignant tumours. Inclusion into this trial is still ongoing and another 18 to 24 months are needed to reach the stipulated group size. A preliminary analysis of survival rate in the test and control groups as well as in the non transfused group can be made

2-3 years after the end of the inclusion. To our knowledge this is the only on-going trial testing the hypothesis that leucocytes in transfusion products are responsible for the immunological effects of transfusion on cancer recurrence.

References

Opelz G., Sengar D.D.S., Micky M.R., Terrasaki P.I. (1973) Effect of blood transfusion on subsequent kidney transplants, *Transplants. Proc.*, 253-259.

Salo M. (1988) Immunosuppressive effects of blood transfusion in anaesthesia and surgery, *Acta Anaest. Scand.* 32 (suppl. 89): 26-34.

Unander A.M. (1992) The role of immunization treatment in recurrent abortion, *Trans. Med. Rev.* 6.

Do Different Additive Solutions have an Influence on the Performance of White Cell Removal Filters?

21 T. Erpenbeck, A. Glaser and W. Mempel

In order to investigate the influence of currently-used additive solutions on the performance of white blood cell (WBC) reduction filters, red blood cells (RBCs) prepared with Optisol and SAG-Mannitol (SAG-M) solution, were filtered using four different WBC reduction filters (LEUCOSTOP 4LT, SEPACELL R-500, SEPACELL R-500 II, PALL RC 400) (Figure 1).

Based on these results, RBCs with PAGGS-Mannitol (PAGGS-M) and Nutricel were filtered using the SEPACELL R-500 II. Units of whole blood were filtered using SEPACELL R-500 II and PALL RC 400 (Figure 2). The buffycoat free RBCs were one to seven days old; the whole blood was one to two days old.

To determine the WBC reduction, prefiltration WBC counts were performed using an automated counter (Sysmex, Toa Medical Electronics Co., Kobe, Japan), and postfiltration WBC counts were measured by a modified flow cytometric method (FACScan, Becton Dickinson GmbH, Heidelberg, Germany).

Results

Figure 1 *Mean white cell reduction rate $\pm SD$ (n = 6)*

	LEUCOSTOP 4LT	SEPACELL R-500	SEPACELL R-500 II	PALL RC 400
Optisol + RBC	96.652% ±2.854%	97.001% ±1.438%	99.726% ±0.172%	99.707% ±0.473%
SAG-M + RBC	99.616% ±0.324%	99.821% ±0.129%	99.964% ±0.026%	99.983% ±0.015%

Overall, highest WBC reduction was obtained using CPDA-1 whole blood.

Filtration of SAG-M RBCs showed the best WBC reduction in each group of tested filters (Figure 1), whereas, Optisol RBCs resulted in the lowest leucocyte depletion rate for all tested filters.

Figure 2 *Mean White Cell Reduction Rate* ±*SD* (n = 6)

	Whole Blood + CPDA-1	RBC + SAG-M	RBC + Nutricel	RBC + PAGGS-M	RBC + Optisol
SEPACELL R-500II	99.995% ±0.002%	99.964% ±0.026%	99.945% ±0.043%	99.923% ±0.106%	99.729% ±0.172
PALL RC 400	99.993% ±0.004%	99.983% ±0.015%	–	–	99.707% ±0.473%

In conclusion the level of white cell depletion in WBC reduced RBCs depends not only on the WBC reduction filter but also on the additive solution used. The presence of platelets and plasma seems to increase the efficiency of both the PALL RC 400 and the SEPACELL R-500 II.

Effectiveness of White Cell Reduction by Filtration with Respect to Blood Storage Time and Blood Product Temperature

22 | A. Glaser, T. Erpenbeck and W. Mempel

Aim

To show a correlation between storage time, blood product temperature and the range of the filter's effectiveness.

Method

Units of whole blood were collected into closed collection sets containing CPDA-1, divided into two equal parts and filtered in 7 different groups (A-G). Filtration was performed using Leucostop LT (Miramed, Mirandola, Italy).

Investigation of the influence of storage time

One half was filtered immediately (6 min) after donation (A_1, B_1, C_1), the other after various storage times. For durations of 30 min (A_2), 2h (B_2) and 12 h (C_2) the blood was held at room temperature. For durations of 24 h (D_1) and 48 h (D_2), the blood was held at 4°C.

In addition, we investigated the filter's effectiveness using various combinations of storage time (6 min/2 h), storage temperature (4°C/23°C/37°C), and surrounding temperature during the filtration process (4°C/23°C) (E-G). Prefiltration counts were performed using an automated counter and postfiltration WBC counts were determined using a flow cytometric method.

Results

1. After a minimum storage time of two hours constant WBC reduction rates are reached, whereas the WBC reduction rates are widely scattered when blood is filtered immediately after donation.

2. These scattered reduction rates can be improved if blood is cooled down after donation for 15 min (E_2).

3. An adverse effect of higher temperatures ($>23°C$) on the capability of the filter used can be seen. However the best reduction rate was achieved by storing the blood for at least two hours without a significant difference between storage at $4°C$ and room temperature (B_2, F_1).

	Storage time (h)	Reduction rate (%)			Storage time (h)	Redution rate (%)	
		Mean±SD	Range			Mean±SD	Range
A_1	0.1	98.10±2.80	92.64-99.96	A_2	0.5	99.74±0.45	98.83-99.95
B_1	0.1	98.82±2.40	94.51-99.92	B_2	2.0	99.97±0.00	99.96-99.97
C_1	0.1	98.96±2.01	95.36-99.92	C_2	12.0	99.95±0.06	99.84-99.98
D_1	24.0	99.87±0.10	99.74-99.97	D_2	48.0	99.83±0.10	99.69-99.95
	Storage time (h); Blood product temperature				Storage time (h); Blood product temperature		
E_1	0.1/23°C	99.13±0.68	98.24-99.96	E_2	0.1/4°C	99.57±0.23	99.26-99.96
F_1	2.0/23°C	99.97±0.03	99.93-99.99	F_2	2.0/37°C	99.75±0.30	99.23-99.98
G_1	2.0/4°C	99.80±0.17	99.54-99.96	G_2	2.0/23°C	99.92±0.11	99.73-99.98

* filtered at constant 4°C; (n=5)

High Efficiency Leucocyte Depletion of Platelet Concentrates using the SEPACELL® PL 5 II BT1 without Flow Reduction

E. Richter, M. Lindner, R. Ullrich, B. Iber, D. Raske,
M. Kerowgan and S.F. Goldmann

23

Alloimmunisation against HLA-antigens is an undesirable result of contaminating leucocytes transmitted to the patient by red cell and platelet transfusions. Leucocyte depletion therefore, is necessary to reduce alloimmunisation and the risk of CMV transmission (Eernisse and Brand 1981, Gilbert et al. 1989) or to prevent non-haemolytic febrile transfusion reactions (NHFTRs) (Sirchia et al. 1990) in multiply transfused patients.

Patients receiving platelet transfusions are usually multiply transfused patients. Therefore, all platelet concentrates (PCs) administered to these patients should be white cell depleted, either at the bed-side or in the blood bank unit (Richter et al. 1993). Until now it has only been possible to perform leucocyte depletion of PCs under conditions of controlled, low flow rates, which for bed-side filtration presents no difficulty. However, in the laboratory, low flow rates are less desirable.

We studied blood bank filtration of PCs using the Asahi SEPACELL® platelet filter PL 5 II N under gravity filtration.

Materials and methods

Random donor PCs were derived from standard laboratory buffy coat production according to normal blood bank routine. Five PCs were pooled prior to filtration.

Additionally, single donor apheresis PCs were obtained.

Both Random donor PCs and Single donor PCs were leucocyte depleted using SEPACELL® PL 5 II BT1 system (Diamed Transfusionstechnik GmbH, Köln, Germany). The PCs were filtered under gravity flow without flow reduction.

We measured platelet recovery (Coulter T-540, Coulter Hialeh) and the residual white cell count (Nageotte chamber, 1/10 dilution).

Results

	Random Donor PCs (n = 10)	Single Donor PCs (n = 5)
Filtration Time (min.)	4.1 ± 0.6	4.2 ± 0.4
Volume (ml)		
- initial	417.6 ± 20.2	220.7 ± 16.0
- after filtration	391.0 ± 14.1	196.7 ± 24.0
Platelet Recovery (%)		
- no saline flush	87	81
Platelet Count		
- initial (Gpt/l)	877.6 ± 117.2	1,208.8 ± 209.6
- absolute	3.7×10^{11}	2.7×10^{11}
Platelet Count		
- after filtration (Gpt/l)	817.8 ± 112.7	1,041.5 ± 194.1
- absolute	3.2×10^{11}	2.2×10^{11}
WBC Count		
- before filtration (Gpt/l)	0.05 ± 0.05	-
- absolute	2.0×10^7	1.6×10^7
WBC Count		
- after filtration (absolute)	$< 0.3 \times 10^6$	0.7×10^6

Discussion

Repeated platelet transfusions of PCs with less than the CILL level (critical immunogenic leucocyte load, Claas et al. 1981) of 1×10^6 leucocytes have been shown to result in reduced alloimmunisation (Van Marwijk Kooy et al. 1991, Meryman et al. 1993).

All filtered PCs were effectively leucocyte depleted as the residual leucocyte counts in all cases, were well below this CILL level.

These results suggest that there is no need to reduce the flow rate when filtering PCs to achieve high leucocyte depletion using the SEPACELL® PL 5 II BT1 system.

In addition, modification of the BT1 configuration by removal of the drip chamber will permit significantly higher platelet recovery in future.

References

Claas F.H.J. et al. (1981) Alloimmunisation against the MHC antigens after platelet transfusions is due to contaminating leucocytes in the platelet suspension, *Exp. Hematol.* 9: 84-89.

Eernisse J.G., Brand A. (1981) Prevention of platelet refractoriness due to HLA antibodies by administration of leucocyte-poor blood components, *Exp. Hematol.* 9: 77-83.

Gilbert G.L. et al. (1989) Prevention of transfusion - acquired cytomegalovirus infection in infants by blood filtration to remove leucocytes, *Lancet* 1: 1228-1231.

Meryman H.T. et al. (1993) The effects of leucocyte depletion on alloimmunisation by platelet transfusions, in Sekigushi S. (ed.) *Clinical Application of Leucocyte Depletion*, Blackwell Scientific publications, Oxford, pp. 173-180.

Richter E. et al. (1993) Leucocyte depletion of red cell and platelet concentrates: clinical importance to patients awaiting organ transplantation, in Sekiguchi S. (ed.) *Clinical Application of Leucocyte Depletion*, Blackwell Scientific publications, Oxford, pp. 183-192.

Sirchia G. et al. (1990) Leucocyte-depleted red blood cells for Transfusion, in Kurtz S.R., Baldwin M.L., Sirchia G. (eds.) *Controversies in Transfusion Medicine*, American Association of Blood Banks, Arlington, pp. 1-12.

Van Marwijk Kooy M. et al. (1991) Use of leucocyte-depleted platelet concentrates for the prevention of refractoriness and primary HLA-alloimmunisation: A prospective randomised trial, *Blood* 77: 201-209.

Evaluation of Two New High Performance Leucocyte Removal Filters (ASAHI PLS-5A PLS-10A) for Use with Platelet Components

24 | V. Sakalas and E. Love

Introduction

There has been over recent years a continual drive to lower the level of residual leucocytes in Blood and Blood Components. This has lead to the production of high performance filters, and with this the need to have a validated method for counting the residual leucocytes.

Along with the production of these leucodepleted components have come new guidelines. Currently within the United Kingdom, guidelines have been produced by the UK/BTS/NIBSC - 'Guidelines for the Blood Transfusion Service 1993'. These guidelines specify that for leucodepleted platelet components the level of Residual leucocytes should be $<1.0 \times 10^6$ per 55×10^9/Platelets.

Also at a consensus meeting in Edinburgh during March 1993, a report was produced to help standardise the use of leucodepleted components and how they are processed and validated. The Consensus stated that levels below 5×10^6 leucocytes per platelet dose were indicated to reduce NHFR due to HLA antigens.

As filters become more efficient and remove larger quantities of leucocytes it becomes more difficult to technically validate the effectiveness of the filters. Routine haematology analysers and standard manual counting techniques are not accurate at such low levels of leucocyte content.

The two new filters evaluated were from the ASAHI Medical Co Ltd. The first filter assessed was the PLS-5A leucocyte removal filter which is suitable for use with 5-7 random platelet units or equivalent Apheresis components. The second filter was the PLS-10A leucocyte removal filter which is suitable for use with 7-12 random donor platelets or the equivalent Apheresis components.

These filters are both designed for use at the bedside. The mechanics and handling of the filters has been fully assessed at the Manchester Royal Infirmary and there were no problems highlighted.

Procedure

The platelet components used were random donor platelets produced using the standard protocol for platelet preparation within the Manchester Transfusion Centre. This consists of a first spin at 3000 RPM for 2.5 minutes to collect platelet rich plasma, followed by a second spin of 3,600 RPM for 13.5 minutes to produce a platelet concentrate with a volume of plasma ranging from 40-60 ml.

The platelets were prepared in a Sorvall RC 3C centrifuge with a H6000A rotor head.

The platelet components were then stored in a rotator sited in a platelet incubator. The temperature was maintained at between 20-24°C during storage. The platelet component used for the evaluation ranged in age from 2 to 6 days.

The platelet components were pooled ensuring they were ABO compatible. Once the platelets had been pooled they were filtered immediately.

The pools ranged in size from 4 to 7 units for the PLS-5A filter and from 8 to 10 units for the PLS-10A filter.

The pooled platelets were filtered without the filter being primed with saline. The rate of filtration was controlled and ranged from 5 to 17 ml per minute.

At the end of the filtration procedure the system was *not* flushed with saline.

Materials and tests

The following tests and assessments were performed on both the Pre and Post filtration samples.

- Platelet Count
- Leucocyte Count
- pH
- Hypotonic Stress Reaction
- Mean Platelet Volume
- Weight

The platelet counts were performed on a SYSMEX K1000 Haematology Analyser. This machine has been validated for platelet counts up to $1800 \times 10^9/L$. The MPV was also assessed on the K1000.

The leucocyte counts were performed on a flow cytometer (ORTHO CYTORON ABSOLUTE), the protocol used was based on the method developed by Bodensteiner (1989) and Dzik et al. (1990). The method is based on the use of propidium iodine to label the DNA within the leucocyte nucleus. These leucocytes will then fluoresce within the flow cytometer system and specifically highlight the leucocytes.

Statistical analysis was performed using NWA Quality Analyst software package.

Results

PLS-5A

The results of the tests performed are displayed in Table 1. The average platelet recovery was 81%. The residual leucocyte count per pack for each pool filtered was $<5.0 \times 10^6$. When comparing the results to the UKBTS 1993 guidelines for leucodepletion of platelet components (Table 2) all the pools filtered had leucocyte counts $<1 \times 10^6$ per 55×10^9/platelets.

PLS-10A

The results of the tests performed are displayed in Table 3. The average platelet recovery was 86%. 7 filters were assessed during the trial, all the platelet components post filtration had leucocyte counts $<5 \times 10^6$/pool. When comparing the results to the UKBTS guidelines for leucodepletion of platelet components (Table 4) all components filtered had residual leucocyte count of $<1 \times 10^6$ per 55×10^9 platelets.

The results of the limited viability studies performed on the platelet components pre and post filtration for both filters clearly showed there was no significant difference between pre and post filtration samples for pH, HSR and MPV ($p > 0.05$).

Table 1 *ASAHI platelet filter PLS 5A evaluation*

			Pre filtration			Post filtration			
No of Units	Age (Days)	flow rate (ml/mins)	Weight (g)	Platelet Counts ($\times 10^9$/p)	WBC Count ($\times 10^9$/p)	Weight (g)	Platelet Counts ($\times 10^9$/p)	Platelet Recovery (%)	WBC counts ($\times 10^6$/p)
5	4	5	229	257	0.15	204	185	72	0.36
4	4	7	185	191	0.09	167	153	80	0.07
5	4	13	266	217	0.14	253	172	79	0.76
7	3	12	321	335	0.27	297	273	81	0.50
5	2	15	230	266	0.06	216	235	88	0.14
5	2	14	265	277	0.24	247	235	85	0.60

Table 2 *ASAHI platelet filter PLS 5A evaluation*

No of units	WBC x10^6/p	Platelets x10^9/p	Scale factor per 55x10^9 Platelets	WBC x10^6 per 55x10^9 Platelets
5	0.36	185	3.36	0.10
4	0.07	153	2.78	0.03
5	0.76	172	3.12	0.24
7	0.50	273	4.96	0.09
5	0.14	235	3.90	0.04
5	0.60	235	4.50	0.13

Table 3 *ASAHI platelet filter PLS 10A evaluation*

				Pre filtration			Post filtration		
No of Units	Age (Days)	Flow Rate (ml/mins)	Weight (g)	Platelet Counts (x10^9/p)	WBC count (x10^9/p)	Weight g	Platelet Counts (x10^9/p)	Platelet Recovery (%)	WBC counts (x10^6/p)
10	4	10	503	666	0.49	490	605	91	0.70
9	4	10	421	544	0.43	400	452	83	0.90
10	4	10	484	501	0.38	457	431	86	0.30
8	4	6	352	364	0.22	328	286	78	0.40
10	4	15	471	506	0.61	450	458	91	2.30
10	5	17	510	585	0.71	485	525	83	0.97
10	3	12	455	480	0.57	421	417	87	2.10

Table 4 *ASAHI platelet filter PLS 10A evaluation*

No of Units	WBC x10^6/p	Platelets x10^9/p	Scale Factor per 55x10^9 Platelets	WBC x10^6 per 55x10^9 Platelets
10	0.70	605	11.00	0.06
9	0.90	452	8.20	0.10
10	0.30	431	7.80	0.03
8	0.40	286	5.20	0.08
10	2.30	458	8.30	0.27
10	0.97	525	9.50	0.10
10	2.10	417	7.60	0.27

Discussion

The limited evaluation clearly shows that both these bedside leucocyte filters (PLS-5A and PLS-10A), when assessed under laboratory conditions consistently produced platelet components which meet the current guidelines for leucodepletion.

All the platelet components filtered either by the PLS-5A or PLS-10A achieved levels below $5x10^6$ per unit, which is taken currently as the level required to prevent alloimmunisation to HLA antigens. All the platelet components filtered also fulfilled the requirements of the UKBTS guidelines for leucocyte depleted components $<1.0x10^6$ per $55x10^9$/platelets.

The viability of the platelet components pre and post filtration was measured using pH, H.S.R. and MPV as variables. The results from both filters showed that there was no significant change in any of the parameters pre and post filtration $(p > 0.05)$

Both PLS-5A and PLS-10A were easy to handle and use. Both filters produced platelet components which met the current specifications for leucodepleted platelet components.

References

Bodensteiner (1989) A Flow cytometric technique to accurately measure post filtration white blood cell counts, *Transfusion* 29: 651-653.

Consensus conference (1993) *Leucocyte Depletion of Blood and Blood Components*, Royal College of Physicians Edinburgh, March 1993.

Dzik et al. (1990) Flow cytometric method for counting very low numbers of leucocytes in platelet production, *Vox Sang.* 59: 153-119.

Guidelines for Blood Transfusion Service (1993) UKBTS/NIBSC (second ed.) HMSO.

Leucocyte Depletion of Platelet Concentrates: Is Poor Filtration Recovery Related to Activation/Aggregation States of Platelets?

25 | M.J. Seghatchian, A.H.L. Ip and P. Krailadsiri

Introduction

Leucocytes in platelet concentrates (PC) not only contribute to transfusion reaction, alloimmunisation, and reduced post-transfusion responses but also, in significant amounts, they have a deleterious effect on platelet surface glycoprotein and accelerate the rate of platelet storage lesion (Sloand et al. 1990, Seghatchian et al. 1994).

Evidence suggests that leucocyte removal by double centrifugation is associated with significant loss of larger and haemostatically active subpopulation of platelets. A lower leucocyte content with improvement in salvage of large platelets is achievable using either automated procedures such as Optipress buffy coat and/or apheresis methods, while the lowest levels of leucocyte content can only be achieved through selective WBC filtration procedure.

Concern nevertheless is expressed on the reproducibility of optimal leucocyte removal by filtration, as often the apparent mean platelet volume (MPV) of filtered platelet concentrates varies, even with the use of well-standardised protocols. This could be related to either within batch variability of the filter or the activation states of platelet preparation as activated platelets are adhesive.

In this study we compared the filtration process efficiency of Sepacell-PL5 in two types: pooled buffy coats and Haemonetics apheresis PC, using two new testing approaches which reflect the functional integrity and aggregation states of platelets (Krailadsiri et al. 1994).

Materials and methods

Platelet collection and filtration were carried out according to NLBTC standard protocol. Paired samples (± 30 mM EDTA) was analysed using Technicon H*1 cells analyser. Platelet indices and leucocytes peroxidase and basophil (WBCp/WBCb) were directly taken from the printouts and dPLT and dMPV (the difference between the paired samples) were calculated.

Results

Process efficiency
This was measured by the fall in platelet count and the degree of leucocyte removal for two types of products stored up to 4 days. Approximately 30 ml plasma is lost during filtration bringing the process recovery to 87% and 60% for OptiPool and apheresis respectively. The process efficiency for apheresis product was much lower, even though the degree of leucocyte removal was comparable. The process efficiency was generally improved using 2-3 days stored products (not shown).

Table 1 *Comparative analyses of pre-post filtration: process efficiency*
Keys: PLT x10^9/L; WBC x10^9/L

	Optipress Pools (n = 35)		Apheresis Platelets (n =35)	
	PLT Rec. %	WBC Dep. %	PLT Rec. %	WBC Dep. %
mean±(SD)	96 (10)	99.91 (0.14)	72 (12)	99.90 (0.11)
Range	121-57	100-99.5	91-60	100-99.8

Changes in morphological and functional integrity
On storage platelets undergo slight discoid/spheric conversion, partial disaggregation and fragmentation leading to products having a lower MPV. Leucocyte filtration, usually leads to the removal of the larger platelets, as identified by a drop of (0.1-0.3 fL) in MPV. Occasionally, however MPV of filtered product increases slightly, suggesting release reaction associated with aggregation may have occurred. The functional integrity as measured by the average dMPV of pre/post filtration appear to be identical (with some exceptions) for Optipress product but clearly different for apheresis-PC. The aggregation states as measured by dPLT is clearly different in Optipress product but remaining the same for apheresis PC (as shown in Table 2).

Table 2 *Morphological/functional integrity of pre/post filtration PC*
Keys: PLT x10^9/L; WBC x10^9/L

	Optipress Pools (n=35)					
	MPV (C)		dMPV		dPLT	
	Pre	Post	Pre	Post	Pre	Post
Mean±(SD)	7.5 (0.5)	7.3 (0.4)	0.3 (0.4)	0.4 (0.4)	73 (51)	48 (40)
Range	8.8-6.6	8.2-6.3	1.1-(-0.9)	1.1-(-0.3)	208 (-19)	144-(-6)
	Apheresis Platelets (n=5)					
Mean±(SD)	8.1 (0.5)	8.0 (0.7)	1.3 (0.6)	0.6 (0.5)	91 (86)	93 (41)
Range	8.5-7.3	8.6-6.9	2.0-0.5	1.2-0.1	221-2	130-29

Hyperaggregability/hyperaggregation states could also be identified by the disparity between peroxidase and basophil on a semi quantitative basis (see Table 3).

Table 3 *Hyperaggregability of pre/post filtration PC*
Key: C = citrate; WBC x10^9/L

| | Optipress Pools (n=35) | | | | | |
	Pre WBCpC	Pre WBCbC	Ratio	Post WBCpC	Post WBCbC	Ratio
Mean	0.183	0.156	1.172	0.024	0.005	4.667
SD	0.294	0.173	1.703	0.043	0.010	4.535
Range	1.66-0	0.78-0.01		0.23-1	0.04-0	
	Apheresis Platelets (n=5)					
Mean	0.622	0.020	31.100	0.128	0.050	2.560
SD	0.492	0.070	7.030	0.097	0.101	0.963
Range	1.19-0.09	0.28-0.36		0.25-.010	0.23-0.00	

We have observed that the higher the disparity (expressed as ratio), the greater is the size of aggregates. In this respect the pre filtration apheresis products showing larger aggregates than Optipress product. While the post-filtration products approach towards unity, though occasionally the disparity between peroxidase and basophil increased in post-filtration products, suggesting cellular injury.

Discussion

Several influencing variables such as centrifugation force (speed/time), accuracy of rotor balancing, poor handling of platelet suspension as well as mode of filtration and filter capacity and flow rate of platelet suspension during filtration need to be defined in order to achieve optimum leucocyte removal with consistency. While 10% platelet loss when achieving ≥99% leucocyte removal is acceptable by gravity-induced filtration, occasionally the loss can reach 30-40%. It is often speculated that lack of a standardised filtration protocol and variability within the batch of filters can attribute to this shortcoming. However the variability in the activation states of platelets in concentrate could also contribute to reduced filtration process efficiency. Based on data, presented here, using two different types of products the latter appears to be more likely.

There has been an urgent need to devise a simple and rapid procedure for assessing platelet concentrates. Such a test must fulfil certain criteria to achieve overall acceptability. It must be easy to perform, reliable and relevant and more importantly reflect the morphological/functional integrity of platelets. We believe that the use of our paired sampling protocol (±EDTA) as applied to both pre/post filtered PC can greatly enhance the quality objective helping in the rapid identification of cause for concerns as well as giving confidence to quality of products used for patients. Their use in routine quality control of the filtration process is highly recommended.

References

Sloand E.M., Klein H.G. (1990) Effect of white cells on platelets during storage, *Transfusion* 30: 333-343.

Seghatchian M.J., Bessos H. (1994) Leucocyte in platelet concentrates accelerates the rate of platelet storage lesion, *Transfus. Sci.* 15 (in press).

Seghatchian M.J. (1994) An overview of laboratory and clinical aspects of leucocyte depleted blood components, *Transfus. Sci.* 15 (in press).

Krailadsiri P., Seghatchian M.J. (1994) Effect of filtration, storage and platelet suspension media in platelet indices, *Transfus. Sci.* 15 (in press).

Leucocyte Depletion by Filtration is Associated With Changes in Platelet Aggregation States: A New Diagnostic Approach

26 | M.J. Seghatchian and P. Krailadsiri

Introduction

Evidence is accumulating that platelets in platelet concentrates (PC) can undergo variable degree of shape changes, activation, microvesiculation and fragmentation during leucocyte filtration (Seghatchian 1994). These changes can be easily monitored in a quantitative manner, by evaluating differential changes in platelet indices (PLT, MPV, PDW, PCT) by using the paired sampling protocol (with and without addition of 30 mM EDTA) (Seghatchian et al. 1992). We have previously reported that the difference in MPV of paired sample ($\pm$EDTA), so called dMPV correlates significantly ($r \geq 0.90$) with the results of various new markers of platelet storage lesion (Vickers et al. 1991, Seghatchian et al. 1993), since EDTA also disperses platelet aggregates the measurement of dPLT of paired samples can provide another useful index of variable degrees of reversible platelet clumps (either present or introduced).

Undiluted fresh citrated platelets also undergo spontaneous aggregation (Sp. Agg.) during preanalytical mixing in plastic tubes followed by repeated counting using Technicon H*1 (Seghatchian 1991). This is associated with a drop in platelet count and the concomitant increase in disparity between leucocyte peroxidase and basophil (WBC_p/WBC_b) results (Krailadsiri et al. 1994). These provide a new tool to assess processing-induced subtle changes in platelet aggregation states and hypo/hyperaggregability.

This report deals with the assessment of leucocyte filtration-induced changes in the aggregation states and morphological/functional states of platelets using the above mentioned new diagnostic approaches.

Materials and methods

Platelet concentrates (PC) were prepared according to NLBTC protocol from whole blood in CPDA-1 anticoagulant and Optipress systems. Sepacell platelet filter 5A (ASAHI) is used throughout in this study.

The protocol for paired sampling involves in placing 0.5 ml of undiluted platelet concentrate in a KE/4 EDTA tube, mixing 5 times by inversion first and allowing to rest for exactly one hour at room temperature for optimal swelling and then cell counting. The differences in cellular indices calculated from the relevant values of the paired samples (i.e. $dPLT = PLT_{+EDTA} - PLT_{citrate}$).

Spontaneous aggregation is carried on 2.5-3.0 ml undiluted citrated PC samples placed in a plastic sampling tube. Counting is then carried out, subsequent to continuous mixing on a roller mixer every 2 min. The use of Technicon H*1 for this purpose is recommended as the instrument by virtue of the reagent used fixes platelets before characterising them on the basis of the flow cytometry principle and light scattering at two low and high angles and light absorbance.

Results

Spontaneous aggregation patterns of non-filtered/filtered products
Fresh platelets (less than 48 h), undergo Sp. Agg., during preanalytical mixing. This is associated by a sharp decrease in platelet count (due to clumping) after a lag period of 5-10 minutes, with a concomitant disparity between WBC_p and WBC_b. Figure 1 shows schematic representation of filtration-induced changes in Sp. Agg. pattern. The lag phase as measured by the fall in platelet count and the concomitant increase in misclassified WBCp appear to be the same for both products however the size of aggregates appears to be much larger in non-filtered products as compared to filtered PC of the same origin. It is noteworthy to refer that on prolonged storage Sp. Agg. is dramatically reduced in line with the drop in platelet aggregation response to ADP (not shown).

Figure 1 *Effect of sequential counting on the fall in PLT and concomitant disparity between WBCp/WBCb*

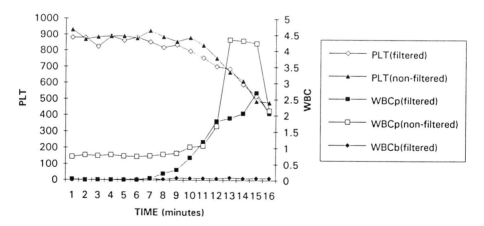

Filtration-induced changes in platelet indices and their response to EDTA
Platelet aggregation states and filtration induced hypo/hyperaggregability can be also monitored qualitatively by changes in MPV of citrated samples and/or quantitatively by dPLT measurement. Upon filtration (n=5) the average MPV of plate-

let found to be reduced by 0.3 fL, with no significant changes in dMPV. The average dPLT value for fresh non-filtered products found to be two fold higher than the average value of dPLT for their filtered counterpart of the same origin. Occasionally, however filtration leads to an increase in dPLT of filtered products and hence poor process efficiency. This occurred more frequently when the product was fresh and more prone to undergo Sp. Agg.

Discussion

Concerns were expressed that leucocyte filtration is associated with the removal of large subpopulation of platelets which are considered to be haemostatically the most active platelet subpopulation (Seghatchian 1994). This is supported experimentally as the MPV of filtered products falls on average by 0.3 fL. However, the fact that post-filtered platelets do still undergo Sp. Agg. at the same rate than its non filtered counterparts is indicative that the observed changes may not be of great significance and possibly the irreversible clumps and/or activated platelets are removed predominantly during the filtration process.

Occasionally however dPLT, which reflect the percentage of aggregated platelets, increases in the post-filtered products, suggesting that cellular injury may occur during additional handling. This shortcoming may be related to activation states of platelet in platelet concentrates rather than the characteristic property of filter itself, though this is not exclusive. We therefore recommend that paired sampling protocol to be applied to both pre and post-filtered products as the essential part of Total Quality Monitoring programme for trends analysis, based on 'diagnostic function testing' than cellular content.

Evaluation of the aggregation states of platelets by automated cell counter, on quantitative basis is simple, accurate, precise and reproducible. In this respect Technicon H*1 system provides an additional advantage over other cell counters for purpose of Sp. Agg. This is due to reagent employed in this system which fixes transient platelet aggregates before characterising them on the basis light scattering at two angles and light absorption properties.

While discoid/spheric and fragmented platelets can easily be differentiated on the basis of their light scattering properties, clumped and aggregated platelets appear in the region 20-200 fL and can be misclassified as pseudoleucocytes and erythrocytes, if no EDTA is used in the sample. This clearly puts in doubt the value of automated cell counters in measuring leucocytes in citrated samples for quality control purpose. The paired sampling protocol (±EDTA), apart from the improved classification of the cellular content has the additional advantage of providing quantitative indications of platelet morphological/functional integrity and aggregation states. Its application, in combination with Sp. Agg., enhances the diagnostic values QC tests for filtered products.

References

Krailadsiri P., Seghatchian M.J. (1994) Effect of filtration, storage and platelet suspension media on platelet indices, *Transfus. Sci.* 15 (in press).

Seghatchian M.J. (1991) An overview of current quality control procedures in platelet storage lesion and transfusion, *Blood Coag. Fibrinol.* 2: 337-360.

Seghatchian M.J., Brozovic B. (1992) An overview of current trends in platelet preparation, storage and transfusion, *Blood Coag. Fibrinol.* 3: 617-620.

Seghatchian M.J., Watts D.C., Laurie A., Savidge G.F. (1993) Platelet storage lesion: changes in the activity state of intra- and extra-cellular von Willebrand factor of therapeutic platelet concentrates, *Platelet* 4: 110-111.

Seghatchian M.J. (1994) International Forum on Leucodepletion: An overview of Laboratory and Clinical Aspects, *Transfus. Sci.* 15 (in press).

Vickers M.V., Ip A.H.L., Cutts M., Tandy N.P., Seghatchian M.J. (1991) Characteristics of platelet concentrates, with particular reference to Autopheresis C Plateletcell: correlation between dMPV and other tests for platelet function, *Blood Coag. Fibrinol.* 2: 361-366.

From Whole Blood to a Leucocyte-depleted Single Component

27 | W. Nussbaumer, W. Hangler and D. Schönitzer

Introduction

For many years, whole blood was transfused after negative result of the infection parameters and of the tolerance test (cross-check). Moreover, much attention has been drawn to the improvment of the blood's security, whether through additional or through improved searching tests or, in case of HIV and HCV, by use of new test procedures.

Only within the last years, the transfusion practice has clearly changed, not only because of a reduction of transfused blood conserves, but there was also detected the additional danger in the transfusion of not needed components of whole blood. Because with each component of whole blood there are not only obtained therapeutic effects, but there are provoked side effects, too.

Also the quality of the single components is much impaired by the storage as whole blood, or there can only be achieved a quality compromise. With that, the basis for the today obligatory component therapy (division in red cells, plasma, platelets, storage under component-specific conditions and therapy with the needed component) has been founded and the therapy with whole blood can be considered as obsolete because of the present state of knowledge.

Filtration procedure

In the use of filter systems, not only the achieved depletion effect, but also the loss of red cells or platelets because of filtration has to be concerned. That is at red cell concentrates, because of the improvement of the filters and of the filtration (ventilation) below 10% and at platelet concentrates according to own research at an average of 12%. We have tested 20 filters of the type Sepacell PL-10 N - Asahi Medical, Tokyo/Krainer Medtechnik, Vienna - (Leucocyte removal filter for platelet concentrates) for their removal rate and have also registered the approximate loss of platelets. The reduction rate was an average of 99.96% and differed between 99.87% and 99.99% .This is equal to an average reduction of log 3.56 at differences between log 2.91 and log 4.33. Each filtered preparation was clearly below the required limit value (CILL) of 5×10^6. The loss of platelets was an average of 12.10% and can be considered as acceptable because the quality improved by filtration. Especially if it is considered, that because of the filtration sensitisation is avoided; therefore numerous platelet transfusions can be saved and the loss of platelets by filtration is compensated. The filters are sold as blood bank filters as well as bed-side filters. Although a filtration at the patient's bed seems to be an elegant method it should be considered, that mainly untrained stuff is handling this and a wrong operation can cause a drastic loss of quality of the endproduct.

Further it is presently concerned to set the time of filtration if possible already at the component production, to remove leucocytes early and to avoid, that during storage metabolic products of disintegrated leucocytes can be released and moreover, the cell fragments cannot be removed by the filters then anymore.

Summary

The transfusion of blood has made great efforts since its establishment in modern medicine. As the component therapy is already undisputed, the leucocyte depletion of blood products is more and more accepted as a further quality improving measure. It was recognised that numerous side effects are caused by the content of leucocytes in the blood components and their removal is obtained by modern filter systems. These are simple in handling and suitable for large amounts in blood banks at the component production as well as directly at the patient's bed as bedside version. Because of integrated ventilation systems, the filters can be drained so that the loss of cells remains minimal. In combination with the meanwhile established component therapy, blood products with a content of leucocyte far below the CILL-value limit can be offered because of the use of these filters and therefore the frequency of leucocyte-specific side effects can be considerably lowered.

Blood Component Separation by a New Gravity Filtration System
Experiences with autologous blood donors awaiting cardiac surgery

28 | U. Taborski and G. Müller-Berghaus

Introduction

Separation of fresh blood units using a hollow fibre filter and gravity flow was first described by Sekiguchi et al. (1990). In addition to fresh plasma (FP), a blood cell concentrate (BCC) was obtained from whole blood (WB). This BCC however, contains all white cells and platelets from the WB. Compared to red cell concentrates (RCCs) produced in the conventional manner, it is less suitable for long term storage. Therefore, Taborski et al. (1993) enclosed a white cell removal filter into this system to obtain white cell and platelet depleted RCCs.

While this previous study was conducted using blood from young, healthy donors, the aim of the current study is to determine whether the process of gravity separation can be used for autologous blood donors with high haematocrit levels, high fibrinogen and high triglyceride concentrations.

Material and methods

Ten white cell removal filters SEPACELL R200 (Asahi Medical Co. Ltd., Tokyo) were sterile docked (SCD, Du Pont) with ten units of the closed blood donation system, ABCC (Diamed Transfusionstechnik GmbH, Köln) comprising a quadruple blood bag and integrated plasma separation filter BCC1 (Asahi Medical Co. Ltd., Tokyo) (Diagram 1). The donor collection bag contained 100 ml CPD solution. 450-500 ml whole blood was taken from each donor. After one hour of storage at room temperature, the blood was separated by gravity flow through the plasma separation filter, into FP and BCC. In using the system, the height differences as shown in Diagram 1 were maintained. Subsequently, the BCC was filtered through the white cell removal filter to obtain a leucocyte and platelet depleted RCC (Diagram 2).

Diagram 1 *Configuration of the ABCC with sterile docked SEPACELL R 200 showing the relative heights of the components during use*

Diagram 2 *Relative heights of the components of the system during the white cell removal process*

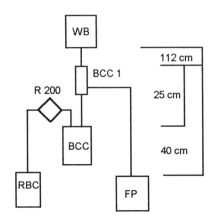

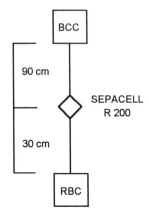

All patients suffered from coronary heart disease and were donating autologous blood for scheduled aortocoronary bypass surgery. All 10 patients were male and aged between 39 and 72 years. The patients were classified into three groups as shown in Figure 1.

Figure 1 *Patient Groups*

Group	Diagnosis	Number (n)
I	Polycythaemia Hct 58.6 ± 7.2 % [53%-60%]	4
II	Hyperfibrinogenaemia cFibrinogen 746 ± 58.3 mg/100 ml [623-955 mg/100 ml]	3
III	Hypertriglyceridaemia cTriglyceride 4147 ± 1588 mg/100 ml [788-11063 mg/100 ml]	3

The filtration times were measured. The obtained WB, BCC and RCC were analysed for volume (Figure 2), haemoglobin content, haematocrit, and blood cell count. The analysis of WB and BCC were carried out on an automatic cell counter (Sysmex CC 180). The white cell counts in the RCCs were measured using a Nageotte chamber (100 μl blood, 900 μl Türks Solution). The platelet counts were measured using a Thoma chamber.

Figure 2 *Volumes of blood components on the day of preparation (ml)*

Patient Group	Whole Blood	BCC	Filtered RCC's	FP	No. (n)
I	571 ± 22	441 ± 17	412 ± 15	166* ± 44	4
II	567 ± 18	404 ± 15	378 ± 4	209 ± 32	3
III	569 ± 24	413 ± 19	385 ± 15	202 ± 25	3
Healthy Donors (Pre study)	559 ± 12	378 ± 10	350 ± 12	205 ± 31	10

* p < 0,05 (I/II, I/III)
BCC: Blood Cell Concentrates
FP: Fresh Plasma

The obtained RCCs were stored at 4°C. In weekly intervals, the haematocrit, potassium ion (K+) concentration in the supernatant (flame photometry), LDL (optimised standard method), lactate (UV test, Boehringer Mannheim), free haemoglobin [modified haemoglobin cyanamide method according to van Kampen, E.J. and Zijistra, W.G. (Boehringer Mannheim)] and pH were measured. The obtained values were not corrected for haematocrit.

All measured parameters were compared with the results of an identical pre-study (Tarborski et al. 1993). The obtained results were statistically reviewed and assessed for significant differences between these two groups (Mann-Whitney-Wilcoxin, U-test, p < 0.05)

Results

Figure 3 shows the results of cell counts of the RCCs on the day of production for all three patient groups. Sample volumes of 10 ml were drawn under sterile conditions from each unit. This has to be taken into account when balancing the overall volumes. The residual volume in the filter and tubing averages about 35 ml. The FP had an average volume of 166 ml (Gp I), 209 ml (Gp II) and 202 ml (Gp III). Only the Group representing patients with high haematocrit levels had a statistically significant reduction of FP volume.

The average filtration times for the gravity separation were 15, 13 and 12 minutes. No difference to the filtration times of the pre-study (Taborski et al. 1993) at 13 ± 3 minutes could be found. The filtration times for leucocyte depletion of all three patient groups were not significantly different to those of the pre-study at 8.4 ± 4.4 min. In addition, the white cell removal was as efficient as in the pre-study. Reductions of 99.96% (Gp I), 99.93% (Gp II) and 99.98% (Gp III) were measured (pre-study 99.95-99.99%). The overall loss of red cell volume in this study was 17% (pre-study: 19%).

Figure 3 *Cell concentration of RCCs on the day of preparation*

Group	Erythrocytes ($10^6/\mu l$)	Platelets (μl^{-1})	Leukocytes (μl^{-1})
I (n=4)	5.66 ± 0.442	3288 ± 417	0.72 ± 0.25
II (n=3)	5.21 ± 0.285	3555 ± 328	0.43 ± 0.19
III (n=3)	5.36 ± 0.300	4201 ± 513	0.58 ± 0.22

Figure 4 shows the results of the long term storage of RCCs over a period of six weeks. In no instance could a statistically significant difference be found between the products of the current patient groups and of the pre-study.

Figure 4 *Long-term storage of RCCs over a period of six weeks*
(Summarised group I to III, n = 10)

	Week 0	Week 1	Week 2	Week 3	Week 4	Week 5	Week 6
Hct (%)	50.2 ± 3.4	50.5 ± 3.8	51.4 ± 3.9	52.3 ± 3.7	52.8 ± 3.8	53.2 ± 3.9	54.1 ± 4.1
LDH (U/l)	55.3 ± 6.2	61.4 ± 7.0	64.8 ± 7.2	68.5 ± 6.5	72.3 ± 7.8	79.4 ± 8.3	88.6 ± 7.2
K^+ (mmol/l)	2.2 ± 0.4	21.4 ± 3.5	23.5 ± 3.2	25.2 ± 4.1	34.6 ± 5.2	38.5 ± 3.9	40.2 ± 5.6
Free Hb (mg/100 ml)	28.6 ± 4.2	35.8 ± 6.2	51.8 ± 7.9	64.6 ± 8.2	77.3 ± 7.1	89.0 ± 8.4	108.5 ± 10.4
pH	7.001	7.013	6.957	6.918	6.853	6.787	6.744

Discussion

This new hollow fibre filter system for gravity separation of whole blood units in conjunction with white cell removal, allows the production of high quality RCCs and FP from a whole blood donation. The exceptionally good quality of the RCCs for long term storage, make this process more suitable for autologous transfusion because autologous RCCs are stored for up to six weeks before transfusion. Therefore, in our opinion, it is extremely important to store RCCs not as BCC but as leucocyte depleted preparations.

The blood components obtained by this gravity separation method however, do not comply with current monographs for standard preparations. This is particularly so in the case of the volumes of FPs. While average FP volumes of 200-220 ml can be obtained from patients with hypertriglyceridaemia and hyperfibrinogenaemia, and from healthy blood donors, from patients with a higher haematocrit, only a reduced plasma volume can be obtained.

In the field of autologous blood transfusion, this is of minor importance. The autologous blood donation product is a single preparation specified for one patient only and as such need not comply with the monograph with respect to volume. Advantages of this overall process compared to non-compliance with the monograph are the high quality of the obtained preparations, the very easy handling of the system and the fact that no centrifuge is required to fractionate the WB unit.

References

Sekiguchi S. et al. (1990) A new type of blood component collector: plasma separation using gravity without any electrical devices, *Vox Sang.* 58: 182-187.
Taborski U. et al. (1993, in press) Blutkomponentenseparation mittels Schwerkraftfiltration: Herstellung eines leukozytendepletierten Erythrozytenkonzentrates, *Z. Infusionsther. Transfusionsmed.*

GEMUSEF Study Group Evaluation of Closed System in-line Filtered Red Cell Concentrates using the SEPACELL INTEGRA® System Performance and Efficiency of the System[*]

29 | N. Müller, E. Richter, G. Matthes and J.G. Kadar

Introduction

White blood cells (WBCs) in red cell concentrates (RCCs) have been claimed to be responsible for numerous side effects of transfusions (Wenz 1990).

With the GMP-controlled production of a blood bag system with integrated filter, containing a widely accepted protein-free storage medium, arose the question of routine applicability of these systems and of the reproducibility of quantitative and qualitative parameters of the resulting blood product.

The purpose of this study is to examine the handling, performance and efficacy of the system in routine blood bank use.

Materials and methods

Whole Blood units were stored for 1-6 hours at ambient temperature prior to processing. The conditions selected for the blood donation and prefiltration processing, including centrifugation of the blood unit together with the in-line filter, are summarised in Figure 1.

In Group 1 and Group 3 the buffy coat (BC) was removed prior to filtration, however, for Groups 2a and 2b, the BC was not removed and only platelet poor plasma was separated. The SAG-M was then transferred through the filter into the RCCs and subsequently the resuspended red cells were filtered. The filtration was undertaken immediately after the centrifugation and within 6 hours of blood donation.

Centrifugation of the system was possible because the centrifuge manufacturing companies, Heraeus and Hettich, developed professional solutions enabling centrifugation of the system using existing equipment.

---

[*] Results are part of the GEMUSEF Study (Berlin, Essen, Köln). This is a German prospective controlled multi-centre study of storage and clinical use of white cell depleted red cell concentrates which have been obtained and processed using the Asahi Medical SEPACELL INTEGRA® system.

Prefiltration cell counts were made using standard automated cell counting techniques. Post filtration white cell counts were made using the high sensitivity Nageotte Chamber.

Figure 1 *Conditions of donation, centrifugation and component separation*

HANDLING	Group 1 (n = 20)	Group 2a (n = 16)	Group 2b (n = 13)	Group 3 (n = 4)
DONATION				
Bag system	DIAMED Transfusionstechnik SEPACELL INTEGRA Top and Bottom bag		DIAMED Transfusionstechnik, SEPACELL INTEGRA 4 x bag conventional	
Max net blood donation (ml)	500	500	450	450
Storage time	min 1 - max 6 hours (after donation and before centrifugation)			
CENTRIFUGATION				
Centrifuge type	Heraeus, Cryofuge 8500		Hettich, Roto Silenta	
Bucket type	6694	6694	4544	4544
Selected g force	3800	3800	2800	2800
Selected plateau time (min)	12	12	10	10
Acceleration score	9	9	9	9
Deceleration score	6	6	6	6
Temperature (°C)	22	22	22	22
SEPARATION OF BLOOD COMPONENTS				
Step 1 (Removing of plasma)	T/B	Manual separation	Manual separation	Manual separation
Step 2 (Removing of Buffy Coat)	Biotrans Separator (selected BC volume of 50 ml)	None	None	Manual separation

Results

Figure 2 shows the leucocyte count pre- and postfiltration for each unit and demonstrates the efficacy of each filtration being without exception, well below the CILL level (5×10^6 leucocytes/unit). Overall, the average post filtration white cell count for the three groups was 0.62×10^5 leucocytes/unit.

Figure 2 *WBC counts in the RCCs - before and after in-line filtration using the SEPA-CELL INTEGRA System*

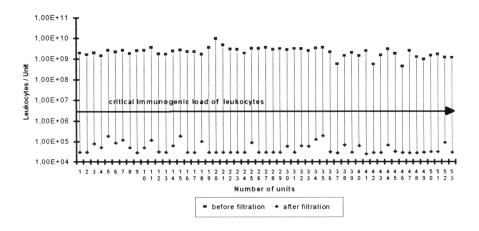

Figure 3 shows the overall results obtained.

There is no significant difference between residual leucocyte counts after filtration regardless of the presence or absence of the BC in the RCCs. The lowest red cell loss (7.2%) was achieved in the RCCs of Group 2. The haematocrits of all RCCs obtained were within the range 59%-63%.

Discussion

The results presented here demonstrate that it is now possible to use a closed, multiple bag system for in-line filtration to produce white cell reduced RCCs of high quality.

The system could be readily implemented for routine use. Some technical problems had to be overcome at the beginning of the investigations, however, the technical solution for the centrifugation of 6 whole blood units per centrifugal step provided by the companies Heraeus and Hettich was appropriate and well functioning. The method of centrifugation can be tailored to the local routine procedure.

The RCCs obtained from blood donations of 450 ml net volume fulfil the quantitative criteria of the quality standard of the European Union (Strassbourg) (>180 g net weight of RCCs/Unit) (*Guide to the preparation...* 1992), however, it should be noted that when two processing steps (BC removal and filtration) are performed, as shown in Figure 3, Group 3, the net weight of red cells resulting from a 450 ml donation does not comply with this standard. Therefore if the BC is removed prior to filtration, it is important to ensure that the initial blood donation volume is large enough to compensate for the loss occurring during processing.

Figure 3 *Results*

Parameters	Group 1 n=20 T/B	p 1/2	Group 2 n=29 with BC	p 2/3	Group 3 n=4 without BC	p 3/1
Filtration time (min) SD	34.25 ± 17.89	n.s.	30.68 ± 16.40	<0.005	26.96 ± 12.07	n.s.
WBC before filtration (x10EE9/l) SD	5.58 ± 2.99	n.s.	9.41 ± 4.17	n.s.	6.65 ± 0.93	n.s.
WBC after filtration (x10E6/l) SD	0.17 ± 0.13	n.s.	0.19 ± 0.15	n.s.	0.18 ± 0.08	n.s.
Red cell content after filtration (x10E12/l) SD	6.67 ± 0.34	n.s.	6.62 ± 0.68	n.s.	6.61 ± 0.30	n.s.
Hct after filtration (%) SD	60.05 ± 2.07	<0.05	59.38 ± 3.09	n.s.	63.50 ± 2.65	<0.05
Red cell loss (through filtration) (%) SD	9.84 ± 2.41	<0.05	7.19 ± 3.55	<0.005	10.73 ± 2.84	n.s.
Weight of SAG-M RCCs after filtration (g) SD	301.70 ± 20.40	<0.05	313.0 ± 20.13	<0.05	264.50 ± 4.93	<0.0005
Plasma weight (g) SD	285.35 ± 17.06	n.s.	266.14 ± 32.07	<0.001	290.00 ± 17.96	n.s.
Net weight of RCCs (g) SD	181.26 ± 15.29	n.s.	186.19 ± 18.90	<0.0005	167.93 ± 6.92	n.s.

The efficiency of the filter enables log 4 reduction of leucocytes (mean residual WBC count/unit = 0.62 x 10^5), irrespective of the initial level of leucocytes (the presence or absence of the BC) in the RCCs. This permits the filter to be integrated within all currently used bag configurations.

The high quality standard which can be achieved using the SEPACELL INTEGRA system is reproducible in different university blood bank centres.

In order to study the parameters of RCCs filtered prior to storage and the clinical effectiveness of the transfusion of such RCCs, a multi-centre study is continuing. (This volume: G. Matthes - 'The Future of Leucocyte Depletion: In-line Filtration'; E. Richter et al. - 'Storage Parameters of the Filtered Red Cell Concentrates' and N. Müller et al. - 'Metabolic Parameters during Storage of the Filtered Red Cell Concentrates')

Acknowledgement

The authors would like to thank the Diamed Transfusionstechnik Study Centre for their initiation of the study and ongoing administrative support.

References

Guide to the Preparation, Use and Quality Assurance of Blood Components (1992) Council of Europe Press, Strasbourg.

Wenz B. (1990) Clinical and laboratory precautions that reduce the adverse reactions, alloimmunisation, infectivity and possibly immunomodulation associated with homologous transfusion, *Transfusion Med. Rev.* 4 (Suppl. 1): 3-7.

GEMUSEF Study Group Evaluation of Closed System in-line Filtered Red Cell Concentrates using the SEPACELL INTEGRA® System Storage Parameters of the Filtered Red Cell Concentrates[*]

30 | E. Richter, G. Matthes, U. Tofoté and E. Rath

White cell depleted red cell concentrates are generally considered to offer the advantages of prevention of non-haemolytic febrile transfusion reactions (NHFTR), reduction of allo-immunisation and prevention of CMV transmission (Sirchia et al. 1990, Pietersz et al. 1993, Gilbert et al. 1989). In current literature leucocyte depleted red cell concentrates are generally considered to be the standard product to administer to immuno-compromised patients or those receiving multiple transfusions.

While degradation of leucocytes during storage leads to release of leucocyte associated virus particles and humoral factors (such as histamine and serotonin) it was proposed by Rawal et al. (1991) that early white cell depletion would be desirable. Early leucocyte depletion within a closed system, is now possible using the Asahi Medical in-line filtration system, SEPACELL INTEGRA®. We studied the handling and efficacy of this system.

Materials and Methods

Whole blood (n = 14) was collected in the SEPACELL INTEGRA® system (Diamed Transfusionstechnik GmbH) comprising quadruple blood bags with integrated Sepacell® filter (Asahi Medical Co. Ltd.). After donation, red cell concentrates (RCCs) were stored at room temperature for approximately one hour and subsequently processed.

We processed according to normal blood bank routine with the exception that centrifugation was performed with special holders (developed by Hettich Zentrifugen), supporting the filter and protecting the blood bags during centrifugation (10 min, 3,000 RPM; ROTOSILENTA, Hettich Zentrifugen).

---

[*] Results are part of the GEMUSEF Study (Berlin, Essen, Köln). This is a German prospective controlled multi-centre study of storage and clinical use of white cell depleted red cell concentrates which have been obtained and processed using the Asahi Medical SEPACELL INTEGRA® System.

After removal of the supernatant plasma, the additive solution (SAG-M) was passed through the filter into the buffy coat containing RCC. Thereafter, the RCC was leucocyte depleted by gravity filtration. The filtered RCC was stored for 35 days at 4°C. Before and after filtration we measured haematological parameters (Coulter CA 560, DILAB) and leucocyte counts using the Nageotte chamber (1/10 dilution in tubes). In addition we tested the following storage parameters: 2,3-DPG (Boehringer), potassium, pH, (LKB, Sweden), pO50 as a marker for oxygen transport capability and oxyhaemoglobin (O_2Hb) (ABL 520, Sweden).

RCCs from routine quality control were used as the control group.

Results and discussion

Figure 1 *Parameters of RBC processing using SEPACELL INTEGRA system*

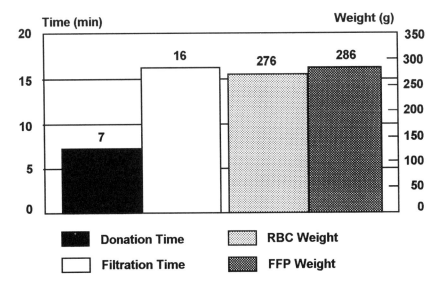

Figure 1 shows the average donation and filtration times (7 min. and 16 min. respectively) and the weights of the obtained plasma and RCCs (286 g and 276 g respectively).

Figure 2 summarises the measured oxyhaemoglobin, 2,3-DPG and pO50 during the storage period.

Filtration of buffy coat containing RCCs, leads to a high volume in the final white cell depleted RCC products. Red cell loss was 8.5%.

All collected FFP's were within the requirements of the German guidelines for blood transfusion (Guidelines 1992).

The residual leucocyte count per unit was $0.6 \pm 0.56 \times 10^5$.

Figure 2 *Storage parameters using SEPACELL INTEGRA system*

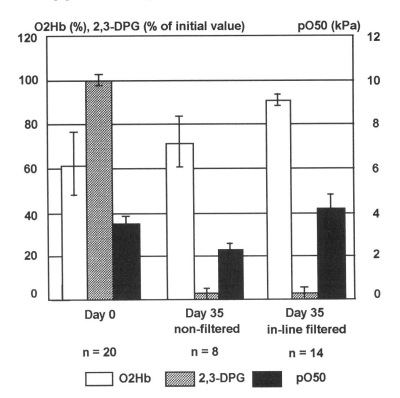

All metabolic parameters during storage were within normal range.

The red cell loss of 8.5% was very low and acceptable.

The white cell removal obtained with this system was as effective as that obtained with log 4 generation filters (Richter et al. 1993). Despite the very high initial leucocyte contamination of the RCCs, white cell counts after filtration were well below the CILL level of 5×10^6.

Compared to unfiltered red cells, in-line filtration prior to storage leads to erythrocytes with high oxygenated haemoglobin (O_2Hb) and, in contrast to the 2,3-DPG loss, to increased pO50 values. We conclude from these findings that this leads to an increased and immediate oxygen transport by the transfused red cells, which should be beneficial for the patient.

Acknowledgement

The authors would like to thank the Diamed Transfusionstechnik Study Centre for their initiation of the study and ongoing administrative support.

References

Gilbert, G.L. et al. (1989) Prevention of transfusion-acquired cytomegalovirus infection in infants by blood filtration to remove leucocytes, *Lancet* 1: 1228-1231.

Guidelines (1992) *Richtlinien zur Blutgruppenbestimmung und Bluttransfusion*, wissenschaftlicher Beirat der Bundesärztekammer des BGA's, überarbeitete Fassung 1991, Köln, Ärzteverlag.

Pietersz R.N.I. et al. (1993) Prestorage leucocyte depletion of blood products in a closed system, *Transfusion Med. Rev. VII*: 17-24.

Rawal B. et al. (1991) Leucocyte filtration removes infectious particulate debris but not free virus derived from experimentally lysed HIV-infected cells, *Vox Sang.* 60: 214-218.

Richter E. et al. (1993) Leucocyte depletion of red cell preparations: Fourth filter generation leads to 4-log reduction. How far can/should we go?, in Smit-Sibinga C.Th., Das P.C., The T.H. (eds.) *Immunology and Blood Transfusion*, Kluwer Academic Publishers, Dordrecht-Boston-London, pp. 121-127.

Sirchia G. et al. (1990) Leucocyte-depleted red blood cells for transfusion, in Kurtz S.R., Baldwin M.L., Sirchia G. (eds.) *Controversies in Transfusion Medicine*, American Association of Blood Banks, Arlington, pp. 1-12.

GEMUSEF Study Group Evaluation of Closed System in-line Filtered Red Cell Concentrates using the SEPACELL INTEGRA® System Metabolic Parameters during Storage of the Filtered Red Cell Concentrates[*]

31 | N. Müller, W. Klimek and J.G. Kadar

Introduction

Bedside filtration of red blood cell concentrates (RCCs) has been shown to be effective for the prevention of febrile non-haemolytic transfusion reactions (FNHTR) (Aubuchon 1988) as well as for the prevention of alloimmunisation in cases of parallel transfusion of other leucocyte depleted blood components (Sniecinski et al. 1988).

Blood bag systems incorporating centrifugable, high efficiency, white cell removal filters are now available which attempt to address the problem of standardising the production of leucocyte depleted RCCs.

This study as part of an ongoing multi-centre evaluation, deals with the storage parameters of leucocyte depleted RCCs obtained using a new blood bag system.

Materials and methods

Twenty whole blood units from healthy donors, were collected in blood bag systems (SEPACELL INTEGRA®, DIAMED Transfusionstechnik GmbH,) comprising quadruple or quintuple blood bags with integrated SEPACELL® filter (Asahi Medical Co. Ltd.). The anticoagulant was CPD, the additive solution was SAG-M.

The upper limit of donation time was set at 15 minutes (Huh et al. 1991). The whole blood units were held at ambient temperature for 4 hours using cooling elements (NPBI, Netherlands), in order to obtain good quality plasma (Pietersz et al. 1989) while maintaining the protective effect of the leucocytes and plasma against initial growth of bacteria (Högman et al. 1991).

---

[*] Results are part of the GEMUSEF Study (Berlin, Essen, Köln). This is a German prospective controlled multi-centre study of storage and clinical use of white cell depleted red cell concentrates which have been obtained and processed using the Asahi Medical SEPACELL INTEGRA® system.

The units were then divided into 3 groups and processed for investigation as follows: Group 1 (n = 10) was separated manually into plasma and buffy coat containing RCCs, after high speed centrifugation (3800 g, 12 minutes at 22°C, Cryofuge 8500, Heraeus Sepatech GmbH, Germany). The RCCs of Group 1 were then in-line filtered in accordance with the manufacturer's instructions to obtain leucocyte depleted RCCs (LD-RCCs). The RCCs of Group 2 (n = 5) were centrifuged as per Group 1 and then buffy coat depleted using a top and bottom system, but not filtered, and served as a control (tb-RCCs). Whole blood (Group 3, n = 5) served as a second control. All blood units were stored for 42 days at between 3-7°C.

The following parameters were determined for all Groups on the day of blood donation (immediately before and after filtration for Group 1) as well as on day 7, 14 and 42.

-   haematocrit
-   red cell, platelet and leucocyte counts (electronic blood particle counter T660, Coulter Electronics GmbH, Krefeld, Germany)
-   Group 1 postfiltration leucocyte count (high sensitivity Nageotte Chamber, Schreck, Hofheim, Germany, diluted 1:10 with Türk's solution
-   free haemoglobin (SIGMA Diagnostics, St Louis, USA) using spectral photometer PM-2, 600 nm wavelength, Zeiss. Oberkochem, Germany);
-   lactate and glucose levels (photometrical assay, Boehringer Mannheim GmbH, Germany)
-   potassium (flame photometer, Eppendorf, Hamburg, Germany)
-   2,3-Diphosphoglycerate (at 365 nm, Boehringer Mannheim GmbH, Germany)
-   O_2-saturation (Ciba Corning, Switzerland)

Results

Figure 1 summarises the results at days 0 and 42 for the metabolic parameters measured in the study. The data shown for Group 1 at day 0 are postfiltration measurements.

Discussion

Lactate and potassium

The potassium levels increased over the storage time and did not differ significantly from the controls.

A higher initial lactate production on day 0 of the RCCs can be observed. To the end of storage, leucocyte depleted RCCs produce less lactate than non-filtered BC depleted RCCs (p < 0.001).

Figure 1 *Summary of results*

Parameter (Unit)	Days	Group 1 LD-RCCs (n=10)	p 1/2	Group 2 tb-RCCs (n=5)	p 2/3	Group 3 WB (n=5)	p 1/3
				Mean±SD			
Free Hb (mg/dl)	Day 0	34.99±14.18	< 0.05	77.36±22.24	n.s.	43.8±28.51	n.s.
	Day 42	111.37±18.17	< 0.01	150.0±0	< 0.001	124.42±6.02	n.s.
Lactate (mmol/l)	Day 0	3.45±0.64	< 0.001	4.66±1.2	< 0.05	1.81±1.13	< 0.05
	Day 42	38.55±1.79	< 0.001	48.58±2.42	< 0.001	28.02±2.84	< 0.001
Glucose (mg/dl)	Day 0	644.22±78.01	n.s.	563.2±56.02	< 0.001	421.2±18.81	< 0.001
	Day 42	292.7±72.04	< 0.01	134.4±22.11	< 0.01	228.6±37.6	n.s.
Potassium (mmol/l)	Day 0	2.0±0	n.s.	2.0±0	< 0.001	3.32±0.33	< 0.00
	Day 42	67.74±18.95	< 0.01	99.84±10.2	< 0.001	48.28±6.06	< 0.05
O₂-Saturation (%)	Day 0	57.26±19.52	n.s.	45.0±27.48	n.s.	38.44±6.47	< 0.05
	Day 42	97.03±0.47	n.s.	94.78±2.75	< 0.001	35.9±3.91	< 0.001
pH	Day 0	7.01±0.03	n.s.	7.04±0.05	n.s.	6.98±0.05	n.s.
	Day 42	6.36±0.03	n.s.	6.33±0.05	< 0.01	6.5±0.07	< 0.05

2,3-DPG
No significant difference could be observed between in-line filtered leucocyte depleted RCCs, unfiltered BC depleted RCCs and WB over the whole storage period. Pietersz et al. (1989) detected significant 2,3-DPG activity differences between filtered and non-filtered RCCs within the first 24 hours of storage but noted however, that these changes are probably due to time differences in sampling rather than filtration.

Free haemoglobin
We found a consistently low haemolysis rate (amount of free haemoglobin) as demonstrated by Matthes et al. (this volume). Our data for the control group of unfiltered RCCs are similar to the literature data (Pietersz et al. 1989). There is apparently no increase of haemolysis due to filtration, $p < 0.001$, (expressed as the amount of free haemoglobin, data not shown here).

During storage we could detect less free haemoglobin in filtered RCCs than in the non-filtered RCCs and whole blood (Figure 2). After 14 days storage the haemolysis rate of the in-line filtered RCCs is significantly lower ($p < 0.05$) than that of the unfiltered RCCs. At 42 days storage haemolysis in the in-line filtered RCCs remains significantly lower than that of the unfiltered RCCs. There is no significant difference between the rate of haemolysis in the RCCs of Group 1 and whole blood (Group 3).

Figure 2 *Free Hb during storage*

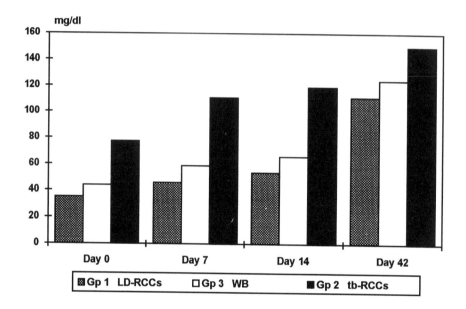

Högman (Högman et al. 1991) demonstrated a decreased haemolysis rate for RCCs in SAG-M over RCCs in CPD and concluded that this resulted from the presence of leucocytes in the RCCs. Depleting the RCCs of leucocytes and then resuspending in SAG-M, revealed no greater haemolysis than when using CPD. Similarly we have found a lower haemolysis rate in the Group 1 filtered RCCs than in the Group 2 unfiltered RCCs, both in SAG-M, and a similar level of haemolysis as for Group 3, Whole Blood, in CPD.

Glucose consumption
After 7, 14 and 42 days of storage, we found less consumption of glucose in leucocyte depleted RCCs (Figure 3) than in either control group. The rate of glucose consumption is graphed as decrease of glucose concentration. This is in line with the results obtained by Pietersz et al. (1989).

O$_2$ saturation
Contrary to Group 3 (WB), in the leucocyte poor RCCs (Group 1) O$_2$ saturation is increasing over storage time (see also Matthes, this volume). The Group 2 BC depleted, non-filtered RCCs demonstrate a similar pattern of improved O$_2$ transport capacity however the changes in absolute numbers are slightly (insignificantly) less pronounced (Figure 4).

Figure 3 *Glucose concentration during storage*

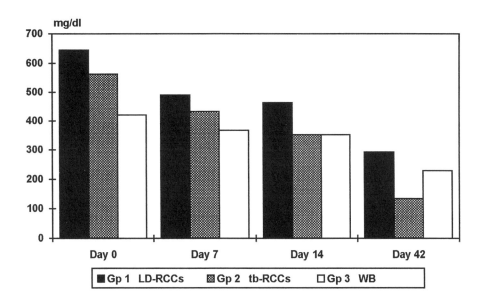

Cell counts
The results for cell content of the filtered RCCs (data not shown in this paper) were consistent with our filtration study (Müller et al., this volume) using the same system.

Haematocrit
The initial haematocrit (%) was measured as follows:

Group 1 - RCCs 58.92±2.13
Group 2 - RCCs 64.06±4.01
Group 3 - WB   38.58±3.62

Conclusion

The non-sterile connection of white cell removal filters to red cell or platelet containing products is handicapped by limited shelf life of the post filtration products (Mac Namara et al. 1984). In this study we concentrated on the metabolic parameters during storage of leucocyte depleted RCCs obtained using a new blood bag system, the SEPACELL INTEGRA®. This system is manufactured incorporating a centrifugable, high efficiency, white cell removal filter into a sterile blood bag configuration eliminating the need for subsequent non-sterile docking of a filter for leucocyte removal.

Figure 4 O₂-saturation during storage

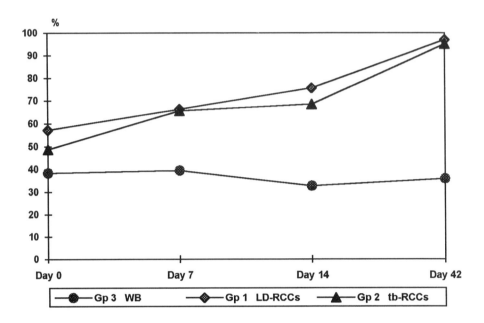

We compared the biochemical parameters of whole blood (CPD), buffy coat depleted non-filtered RCCs (SAG-M) and in-line filtered resuspended leucocyte depleted RCCs (SAG-M) stored for 42 days.

Our results, similarly to the findings of Matthes et al. (this volume), underline the importance and demonstrate the significance of early leucocyte depletion of stored red cell concentrates. The clinical consequences of the optimised metabolic properties still have to be clarified. The first clinical results indicate the potential benefit of these optimised metabolic properties (Matthes, this volume).

The protein poor environment of the filtered RCCs may affect the metabolic activity and immunological characteristics of the red cells during storage. In addition, there may be immunological effects resulting from the filtration process itself. These aspects are undergoing further investigation.

Acknowledgement

The authors would like to thank the Diamed Transfusionstechnik Study Centre for their initiation of the study and ongoing administrative support.

References

Aubuchon, J.P. (1988) Blood centre implications of leucocyte depletion by filtration, in Brozowic B. (ed.) *The Role of Leucocyte Depletion in Blood Transfusion Practice,* Blackwell Scientific, New York, pp. 35-40.

Davey C., Leng Chong S.N., Garcez (1989) Preparation of white cell depleted red cells for 42 day storage using an integral in line filter, *Transfusion* 29: 496-499.

Högman C.F., Eriksson L., Ericson A., Reppucci A.J. (1991) Storage of Saline Adenine Glucose Mannitol suspended red cells in new plastic container: PVC-plasticised with butyryl n trihexyl citrate, *Transfusion* 31: 26-29.

Högman C.F., Gong J., Eriksson L., Hambraeus A., Johansson C.S. (1991) White cells protect donor blood against bacterial contamination, *Transfusion* 31: 620-626.

Huh Y.O., Lichtiger B., Giacco G.G., Guinee V.F., Drewinko B. (1991) Effect of donation time on platelet concentrates and fresh frozen plasma, *Vox Sang.* 56: 21-24.

Mac Namara E., Clarke S., Mc Cann S.R. (1984) Provision of leucocyte poor blood at the bedside, *J. Clin. Path.* 37: 669-672.

Pietersz R.N.I., Steneker, Reesink H.W. (1993) Prestorage leucocyte depletion of blood products in a closed System, *Transfusion Med. Rev.* 7: 17-24.

Pietersz R.N.I., De Korte D., Reesink H.W., Dekker W.J.A., Van den Ende A., Loos J.A. (1989) Storage of whole blood for up to 24 hours at ambient temperature prior to component preparation, *Vox Sang.* 56: 145-150.

Sniecinski I., O'Donnel M.R., Nowicki B., Hill L.R. (1988) *Blood* 71: 1402-1407.

Preparation of Leucocyte Depleted Red Blood Cell Concentrates Using Optipac Bloodbags With Integral Filter

32 R. Beltzig, P. Lambert and V. Thierbach

Introduction

Leucocytes in blood components can lead to numerous immunological effects (Myllylä 1993) and, due to leucocyte - associated viruses, can transfer infections associated with transfusion (Rawal et al. 1990).

Most leucocyte depleted red blood cell concentrates (RCC) are used for patients with oncological or hematological disorders.

Currently the filtration of a RCC is done on demand. For this purpose RCC, buffy coat removed are prepared in the traditional Optipac blood bag system and stored for up to 10 days. The leucocyte filter is connected using a sterile technique.

The new Optipac blood bag system with integral filter was evaluated for suitability in routine use and the effectivity of prestorage filtration of RCCs was investigated.

Material and methods: the blood bag system

Figure 1 *Optipac with integral Sepacell R 2000 Filter*

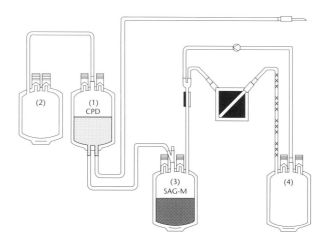

The new Optipac System (by Baxter) consists of a primary bag (Council of Europe 1992) with bottom and top outlet ports and is filled with 63 ml of CPD. The top outlet port leads to an empty 400 ml bag (Davey et al. 1989) for the reception of the plasma. One outlet port on the bottom leads to the venous cannula via a blood sampling tube. The second port on the bottom leads to a bag with 100 ml of SAG-M (Myllylä 1993). This bag is connected with a Sepacell R 2000 Filter and a 450 ml empty bag (Rawal et al. 1990) for reception of leucocyte-depleted red blood cells (Figure 1).

Production of blood components

The centrifugation of 450 ml of whole blood was performed in a Hettich Roto Silenta RP (Hettich, Tuttlingen) in double chamber centrifuge bucket No. 4560 with integrated filter holder.

Using an Optipress the blood is then separated in plasma and buffy coat depleted red cell concentrate. Following a storage period of 20-24 hours at 2-6°C a gravity filtration of the RCC was performed. After completion of the filtration the sterile air was pressed into the upper bag via the bypass. This leads to a maximum yield of erythrocytes.

Cell count

The cells were counted using a Coulter T660 and the leucocyte content of the filtered RCC was determined with a Nageotte hemocytometer.

Determination of hemoglobin

In 8 units of leucodepleted RCC the free hemoglobin in the supernatant was determined with spectrophotometry at 546 and 680 nm.

Results: erythrocyte concentrate

The mean erythrocyte content per RCC (n=31) prior to filtration was $1.79 \pm 0.18 \times 10E12$ and following filtration was $1.59 \pm 0.20 \times 10E12$.

The mean leucocyte content prior to filtration was $1.08 \pm 0.45 \times 10E9$ and following filtration was $0.19 \pm 0.08 \times 10E6$.

The mean extracellular hemoglobin on the 35th day of storage was 47.2 μmol/l.

Handling of blood bag systems

After training of the users, the system was safe and handling was easy.

Discussion

Using the new Optipac blood bag system leucocyte depleted erythrocyte concentrates can be prepared successfully in a closed system under standardized conditions. Integration of the filtration process in daily routine is easier using the new procedure. Filtered RCC can be stored safely during the maximum storage period. Prestorage filtration prevents the decay and release of cellular substances of leucocytes (Davey et al. 1989). In each case the leucocyte content of the filtered RCC was less than 0.8 x 10E6 and thus less than a sixth of the required limit of 5 x 10E6 leucocytes per RCC (Council of Europe).

References

Council of Europe (1992) *Guide to the Preperation, Use and Quality Assurance of Blood Components*, p. 63.

Davey R.J., Carmen R.A., Simon T.L. (1989) *Transfusion* 29: 456-499.

Myllylä G. (1993) Abstracts of consensus conference 'Leucodepletion of blood and blood products', Edinburgh.

Rawal B.D., Davis R.E., Busch M.P., Vygas G.N. (1990) *Transfusion Med. Rev.* 4 (f1): 36-41.

Leucocyte Depletion of Red Cell Concentrates Evaluation of Conventional Filters and a Closed In-line System

D. Barz, K. Stange, D. Staack, R. Lehmann and
K. Schnurstein

33

In order to prevent alloimmunization in chronically transfused patients, transfusion of leucocyte depleted blood products is generally indicated.

However, the assumption that filtered blood products can prevent alloimmunization has not been confirmed in all cases. Filtered blood products can only prevent a primary immune-response. Previously transfused or immunised patients show, even with the use of leucocyte depleted blood products, a secondary immune-response and produce HLA- or platelet-specific antibodies.

Using leucocyte depleted red cell concentrates (LD-RCCs), the production of antibodies can be reduced, however, our own investigations have shown that some chronically transfused patients developed cytotoxic HLA- and platelet-antibodies even when receiving LD-RCCs and white cell depleted platelet concentrates (LD-PCs). The incidence is greater in female patients (according to our evaluations > 10%) due to pregnancy, the consequence of which is an increased tendency to antibody production. Male patients show a much lower incidence of antibody formation (according to our evaluations > 3% of patients).

An explanation for such antibody production could be the passage of HLA-bearing cell structures (intact leucocytes and platelets and even HLA-bearing fragments) through the filter. Determining whether there is a passage of HLA bearing cell fragments through currently available white cell removal filters was a principle feature of this study.

Material and methods

The following commercial filter systems, PALL BPF 4 BBS (PALL, Dreieich), ASAHI SEPACELL RS 200 B1 (DIAMED TRANSFUSIONSTECHNIK, Köln), and NPBI Cellselect (BIOTRANS, Dreieich) were used for filtration of buffy coat poor red cell concentrates (RCCs), produced under routine conditions and stored prior to filtration.

The RCCs were stored at 4°C for different storage times. Cell-counting of HLA-Class I and II antigen bearing cells (leucocytes, platelets) and cell fragments, before and after filtration with each of the filter systems, was carried out.

We also evaluated a new, closed blood bag system with incorporated white cell removal filter, SEPACELL INTEGRA (DIAMED TRANSFUSIONSTECHNIK, Köln), and compared it to the previously mentioned filters. Whole blood was stored at room temperature for 2 hours after donation and then separated into components. After removal of plasma and buffy coat, the RCCs were filtered within this system. Samples were examined before and after filtration as for the conventional filters.

The cell counts were measured using an automated cell counter (Coulter Electronics GmbH, Krefeld), the Neubauer chamber (for platelets) and the Nageotte chamber (for leucocytes). The detection limit of this latter method is acknowledged as 0.3×10^5 leucocytes/unit.

For the detection of antigen bearing cell ghosts (membrane-particles) we used a modification of the MAIPA-assay (Monoclonal Antibody Immobilisation of Platelets or Platelet Antigen) (Kiefel et al. 1987).

Briefly the HLA Class I or II bearing cells or cell fragments are detected by preincubation with human serum (obtained from immunised patients having multispecific HLA alloantibodies) and subsequently with a second, Monoclonal mouse anti-human antibody (DIANOVA, Hamburg, Germany). After washing, cells are solubilised and centrifuged at low temperature. The cell Lysate is diluted and transferred to a microtiter plate with wells precoated with goat-anti-mouse IgG. The immobilised, mouse anti human MoAb-human alloanti-IgG-HLA Class I or II antigen complexes (the latter derived from cells or cell fragments positive for these antigenic properties) are detected by using GAM-IgG, Monoclonal Antibodies, Peroxidase (DIANOVA, Hamburg, Germany) and OPD (DAKOPATS, Germany). Blood cells or blood cell derived membrane fragments expressing HLA Class I or II antigens are immobilised and detected by this test system increasing the extinction measured photometrically at a wavelength of 490 nm.

According to our previous experience (Barz et al.), the results are regarded as positive when the optical density (OD) exceeds a level of 0.200 units.

Table 1 *Leucocyte and platelet depletion results*

Filter/system	Leucocyte depletion % (mean values)	Platelet depletion % (mean values)
PALL BPF4 BBS	99.998	96.2
SEPACELL RS 200 B1	99.995	93.0
NPBI CELLSELECT	99.998	94.1
SEPACELL INTEGRA	99.998	99.5

Results

The filtration results obtained verified the claimed efficiency of the 4 (log 4) white cell removal filters irrespective of the storage time of the SAG-M resuspended RCCs (Table 1).

Figure 1 *Detection of HLA Class I Antigens before Filtration and after Filtration using the Pall BPF 4 BBS System*

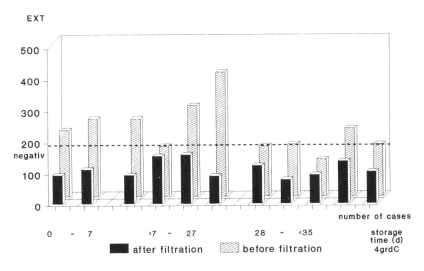

prinzip of the MAIPA-test

Figure 2 *Detection of HLA Class I Antigens before Filtration and after Filtration using the Sepacell RS 200 B1 System*

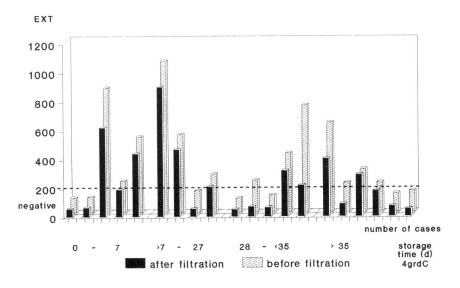

prinzip of the MAIPA-test

Figure 3 *Detection of* HLA *Class I Antigens before Filtration and after Filtration using the Cellselect System*

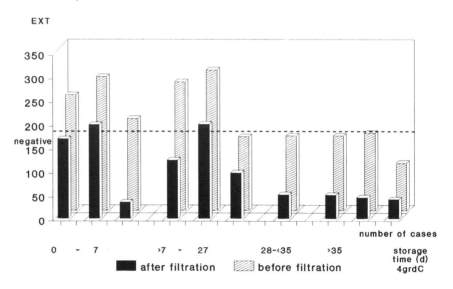

prinzip of the MAIPA-test

Figure 4 *Detection of* HLA *Class I Antigens before Filtration and after Filtration using the Sepacell Integra System*

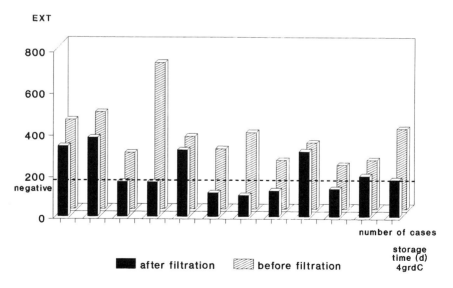

prinzip of the MAIPA-test

The average leucocyte content post filtration did not differ between the investigated filters.

Figures 1, 2, 3 and 4 demonstrate the results obtained by using the modified MAIPA assay with HLA-Class I specificity.

The average ability of the three conventional filters to reduce HLA-antigen containing material seems to be equal for each filter tested (0.100 to 0.150 OD Units/filtration).

For the in-line system there is a tendency to increasing effectiveness, expressed by pre/post extinction differences of 0.200-0.300 OD Units/filtration.

Discussion

The leucocyte depletion by all tested filters was > 99,99%.

HLA-Class II antigen bearing cells could not be detected in any sample after filtration.

The results of the study point out that as storage time at 4°C increases, the antigenicity (e.g. HLA-Class I) decreases.

In RCCs stored for > 28 days, we could detect before filtration, HLA-Class I antigen bearing cells in 6 out of 20 cases (30%). In comparison to RCCs stored < 22 days we could detect HLA-Class I antigen bearing cells in 15 out of 21 cases (71%) before filtration.

Saarinen et al. (1993) could demonstrate that alloimmunisation could be completely prevented using freshly filtered blood components, however the exact time of filtration after blood donation has not been specified by the authors.

Ramos (1994) found white cell fragments to be detectable after filtration of platelet concentrates using polyester fibre filters of the third generation. In order to evaluate the quality of the filtered blood products, there should be an evaluation of cell fragments in addition to chamber counting.

This study addressed the parallel detection of HLA-antigen bearing cell fragments in addition to the leucocyte content of filtrated RCCs. We demonstrated the overall effectiveness of all filters evaluated for the removal of intact white blood cells and platelets from red blood cell concentrates held for different storage times. The remaining HLA-Class I antigenicity of the filtrated RCCs is directly related to the inability of the filter to retain cell fragments.

References

Barz D., Gossrau E., Witt-Meise T. (in press) Nachweis von antigenen Substanzen in verschiedenen aufbereiteten Plasmapräparaten, *Beiträge zur Infusionstherapie* 32.

Kiefel V., Santoso S., Weisheit M., Mueller-Eckhardt C. (1987) Monoclonal antibody-specific immobilization of platelet antigenes (MAIPA): A new tool for the identification of platelet-reactive antibodies, *Blood* 70: 1722-1726.

Ramos R.R., Curtis B.R., Duffy B.F., Chaplin H. (1994) Low retention of white cell fragments by polyester fiber white cell-reduction platelet filters, *Transfusion* 34: 31-34.

Saarinen U.M., Koskimies S., Myllylä G. (1993) Systematic use of leukocyte-free blood compo-
    nents to prevent alloimmunization and platelet refractoriness in multitransfused children
    with cancer, *Vox Sang.* 65: 286-292.

List of Authors

Andreu, Professor G.
Hotel Dieu, Poste de Transfusion Sanguine, 1 Place du Parvis Notre Dame, 75181 Paris Cedex 4, France

Berlin, Dr. Gösta
The Department of Transfusion Medicine, University Hospital, S-58185 Linköping, Sweden

Böck, Dr. M.
Medizinische Akademie Magdeburg, Institut für Blutspende und Transfusionswesen, Leipziger Strasse 44, 39120 Magdeburg, Germany

Brozović, Dr. B.
Tawam Hospital, Al Ain, Abu Dhabi, U.A.E.

Brand, Dr. Anneke
Department of Immunohaematology/Blood Bank, University Hospital, Rijnsburgerweg 10, 2333 AA Leiden, The Netherlands

Dzik, Dr. W.H.
Director Blood Bank and Tissue Typing, New England Deaconess Hospital, 185 Pilgrim Road, Boston MA 02215, USA

Högman, Professor Claes F.
Department of Clinical Immunology and Transfusion Medicine, University Hospital, S-75185 Uppsala, Sweden

Meryman MD, Dr. Harold T.
Head, Transplantation Dept., Holland Laboratory, 15601 Crabbe Branch Way, Rockville, MD 20855, USA

Masse, Mr. Maurice
Centre Regional de Transfusion Sanguine, 1 Boulevard Fleming, B.P. 1937, 25020 Besançon, Cedex France

Matthes, Prof. Gert
Universitätsklinikum Charité, Institut für Transfusionsmedezin, Schumannstrasse 20/21, D-10098 Berlin, Germany

Nishimura, Dr. T.
Research and Development Laboratory, Asahi Medial Co Ltd, 2111-1 Oaza-Sato, Oita city, Oita 870-03, Japan

Parrott, Mr. Neil R.
Department of Surgery, Manchester Royal Infirmary, Oxford Road, Manchester M 13 9WH, UK

Rivers, Dr. Rodney
Reader in Neonatal Medicine, St Mary's Hospital Medical School, The Queen Mother Wing, St Mary's Hospital, South Warf Road, London W2 1NY, UK

Sekiguchi MD, Dr. Sadayoshi
Director, Hokkaido Red Cross Blood Center, Yamanote 2-2, Nishi-Ku, Sapporo 063, Japan

Sirchia MD, Professor G.
Director, Centro Trasfusionale e di imunologia dei Trapianti, via Francesco Sforza 35, Milano, Italy

Addresses of poster presenters

Barz, D., K. Stange, D. Staack, R. Lehmann, K. Schnurstein
Department of Transfusion Medicine, Clinic for Internal Medicine, University of Rostock, Rostock, Germany

Beltzig, R., V. Thierbach
Universität Leipzig, Institut für Transfusionsmedizin, Leipzig, Germany

Erpenbeck, T., A. Glaser, W. Mempel
Transfusion Centre, III Medical Department, Klinikum Großhadern, University of Munich, München, Germany

Garritsen H.S.P., P. Krakowitzky, K. Härtel, K. Lippert, C. Schneider, W. Sibrowski
Department of Blood Transfusion and Transplantation Immunology, University Hospital Münster, Münster, Germany

Glaser, A., T. Erpenbeck, W. Mempel
Ludwig-Maximillans-Universität München, Klinikum Großhadern, Transfusions-zentrum/Med. III, München, Germany

Haglind, E.
Department of Surgery, Sahlgrens University Hospital, S-413 Göteborg, Sweden

Kadar, J.G.
Blood Bank and Immunohaematology, Medical School Hannover, Germany

Klimek, W.
Institute of Transfusion Medicine, University Clinic, Essen, Germany

Knutson, F, C.F. Högman
Department of Clinical Immunology & Transfusion Medicine, University Hospital, S-75185 Uppsala, Sweden

Krailadsiri, P.
National Blood Centre, Bangkok, Thailand

Lambert, P.
Baxter Deutschland GmbH, Fenwal Division, Edisonstrasse 3-4, Postfach 1165, D-85701 Unterschleissheim, Munich, Germany

Müller, N.
Institute of Transfusion Medicine, University Clinic Essen, Germany

Nussbaumer, W., W. Hangler, D. Schönitzer
Department of Immunology and Blood Bank, University Hospital, Innsbruck, Austria

Richter, E.
Institute of Transfusion Medicine, University Clinic Charité, Medical Faculty, Humboldt University, Berlin, Germany

Richter, E., M. Lindner, R. Ullrich, B. Iber, D. Raske, M. Kerowgan, S.F. Goldmann
German Red Cross Blood Bank, Baden-Württemberg, Mannheim Institute, Germany

Sakalas, V.F., E.M. Love
Manchester Regional Transfusion Centre, Plymouth Grove, Manchester, England

Seghatchian, M.J., AHL Ip
QA Laboratory, North London Blood Transfusion Centre, Colindale, London

Smeets, F.
Department of Obstetrics and Gynaecology, University Hospital Münster, Münster, Germany

Taborski, U., G. Müller-Berghaus
Max-Planck Institute for Physiological & Clinical Research, Kerckhoff Clinic, Department of Haemostasiology & Transfusion Medicine, Bad Nauheim, Germany

Takahashi, T., H. Abe, M. Hosoda
Hokkaido Red Cross Blood Centre, Sapporo, Japan

Takahashi, T., S. Nakajo, S. Chiba, M. Hosoda
Hokkaido Red Cross Blood Centre, Sapporo, Japan

Tofoté, U., E. Rath
Institute for Transfusion Medicine, University Clinic Charité, Medical Faculty, Humboldt University, Berlin, Germany

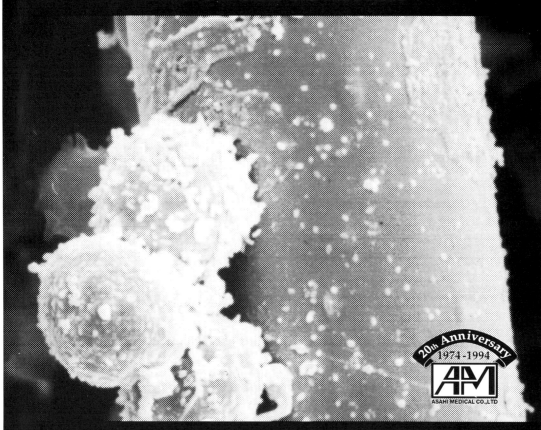
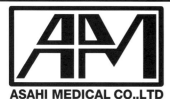